This volume aims to unravel the step-by-step processes that result in colorectal cancer – one of the commoner causes of death in the Western world. Advances in our scientific understanding of the disease suggest that there is a clear progression of events leading to localised malignancy. It thus provides an excellent model for the study of carcinogenesis. The volume draws together some of the epidemiological, clinical and scientific factors which help to give a broader understanding of colorectal cancer and, it is hoped, encourage closer collaboration between scientists and clinicians. The volume also emphasises the diagnostic, therapeutic and prognostic advances arising from these developments and highlights other areas where collaboration between scientists and clinicians is needed.

The volume is suitable for all those with a professional scientific or clinical interest in colorectal cancer, including oncologists, cancer research scientists, cancer surgeons and gastroenterologists.

Cambridge Monographs on Cancer Research

Colorectal cancer: a scientific perspective

Cambridge Monographs on Cancer Research

Books in this Series

Martin R. Osborne and Neil T. Crosby *Benzopyrenes*

Maurice M. Coombs and Tarlochan S. Bhatt *Cyclopenta[a]phenanthrenes*

M. S. Newman, B. Tierney and S. Veeraraghavan *The chemistry and biology of benz[a]anthracenes*

Jürgen Jacob *Sulfur analogues of polycyclic aromatic hydrocarbons (thiaarenes)*

John Higginson, Calum S. Muir and Nubia Muñoz *Human cancer: epidemiology and environmental causes*

R. G. Harvey *Polycyclic aromatic hydrocarbons*

W. F. Karcher *Dibenzanthracenes and environmental carcinogenesis*

Anne R. Kinsella *Colorectal cancer*

Forthcoming Volumes

W. Lijinsky *The chemistry and biology of* N-*nitroso compounds*

Valda M. Craddock *Cancer of the esophagus*

Colorectal cancer: a scientific perspective

ANNE R. KINSELLA

Department of Surgery,
University of Liverpool

With the assistance of
PHILIP F. SCHOFIELD

Withington Hospital, Manchester

CAMBRIDGE
UNIVERSITY PRESS

Published by the Press Syndicate of the University of Cambridge
The Pitt Building, Trumpington Street, Cambridge CB2 1RP
40 West 20th Street, New York, NY 10011-4211, USA
10 Stamford Road, Oakleigh, Victoria 3166, Australia

First published 1993

Printed in Great at the University Press, Cambridge

A catalogue record for this book is available from the British Library

Library of Congress cataloguing in publication data

Kinsella, Anne R.
Colorectal cancer: a scientific perspective/Anne R. Kinsella
with Philip F. Schofield.
p. cm.
Includes index.
ISBN 0 521 36199 0 (hardback)
1. Colon (Anatomy) – Cancer. 2. Rectum – Cancer. I. Schofield, P. F.
(Philip F.), 1930 – . II. Title.
[DNLM: 1. Colorectal Neoplasms – etiology. 2. Colorectal
Neoplasms – physiopathology. WI 435 K56c]
RC280.C6K56 1993
616.99′43475 – dc20
DNLM/DLC
for Library of Congress 92–21069 CIP

UP

Contents

Preface

A neoplasm is an abnormal mass of tissue, the growth of which exceeds and is unco-ordinated with that of the normal tissues and which persists in the same excessive manner after cessation of the stimulus which evoked the change. (R. A. Willis, *Pathology of Tumours*, 1948)

Willis's statement defines a group of diseases about which we have an increasing fund of knowledge but areas of ignorance. Malignant neoplasms invade and metastasise, but this facility varies markedly between tumours of different tissues and even between tumours of the same tissue. The reasons for this variation have to be sought at the molecular level but the consequences affect the clinician in day-to-day practice.

Colorectal carcinoma is numerically one of the commoner causes of death in the Western world and for this reason the public have a profound interest in resolving the many imperfections in our understanding which still persist. It is a source of regret that the existing fund of knowledge is not widely available to the professionals who grapple with these problems. The scientist working in molecular biology has made considerable progress in a variety of fields in recent years but is often ignorant of the facts which are well known to clinicians treating patients with colorectal disease. Conversely, most clinicians have only a superficial knowledge or are totally ignorant of the advances made by the scientist.

Some techniques developed in the research laboratory, such as flow cytometry and the use of monoclonal antibodies, have begun to take a place in the prognostic armamentarium of the pathologist. The use of monoclonal antibodies to direct materials to a tumour for diagnostic or therapeutic manipulation has begun to pass to the diagnostic radiologist and the medical oncologist, but the vast majority of the work in molecular biology is, as yet, unappreciated by many clinicians.

In the last decade more detailed investigations of the genome have produced considerable interest, but how this expanding knowledge becomes of value to the patients is not yet certain. We have felt that it is important to encourage direct collaboration between laboratory workers and clinicians managing colorectal patients and have found that by collaboration, understanding increases for both the scientist and the physician. This greater understanding appears likely to make scientific work and clinical care more relevant and speed the path to fuller understanding. The multidisciplinary approach is particularly relevant in colorectal cancer where there is a good knowledge of the pathological, epidemiological and surgical factors. From the scientific point of view, colorectal carcinoma is an ideal system in which to study the multifactorial nature of carcinogenesis because it is a disease with a very obvious step-wise progression from normal through pre-malignant to localised malignant and finally a metastatic stage.

There is evidence of genetic alterations at each of the three transitions. All three transitions have profound therapeutic and prognostic significance. The identity of interest between the molecular biologist and the clinician is obvious. This monograph attempts to assemble some of the factors – epidemiological, clinical and scientific – which would help to give a broader understanding of the subject of colorectal cancer and would hope to encourage scientists and clinicians towards closer collaboration.

Manchester Philip F. Schofield
February 1992

Acknowledgements

The authors would like to acknowledge the help of Dr S. Venitt, ICR, Sutton, Surrey, and Mr B. A. Taylor, Senior Lecturer in Surgery, University of Liverpool, for their critical reading of some of the chapters. They would also like to thank Dr C. Pareskeva for making available preprints of articles.

A. R. K.
P. F. S.

Abbreviations

AMMN	Acetoxymethyl-methylnitrosamine
APC	Adenomatous polyposis coli
AOM	Azoxymethane
BCNU	1,3-bis(2-chloroethyl)-1-nitrosourea
BHA	Butylated hydroxyanisole
BHT	Butylated hydroxytoluene
CEA	Carcino-embryonic antigen
CFS	Cancer family syndrome
CHIRPE	Congenital hypertrophy of the retinal pigmented epithelium
CRC	Colorectal carcinoma
DAS	Diallyl sulphide
DF	Dietary fibre
DFMO	Difluoromethylornithine
DMBA	Dimethylbenzanthracene
DMF	*N*,*N*-dimethylformamide
DMH	1,2-Dimethylhydrazine
FAP	Familial adenomatous polyposis (*see also* FPC and APC)
FPC	Familial polyposis coli (*see also* FAP and APC)
5-FU	5-Fluorouracil
GS	Gardner's syndrome (*see also* FPC and FAP)
GTP	Guanosine triphosphate
HNPCC	Hereditary non-polyposis colorectal cancer (*see also* CFS)
IARC	International Agency for Research on Cancer
IDF	Insoluble dietary fibres
IVT	*In vitro* tetraploidy
Ki-MuSV	Kirsten murine sarcoma virus
MAM	Methyl azoxymethanol acetate
7-MeG	*N*-7-methylguanine

MNNG	*N*-methyl-*N′*-nitro-*N*-nitrosoguanidine
MNU	*N*-methyl-*N*-nitrosourea
ODC	Ornithine decarboxylase
O^6MeG	*O*-6-methylguanine
OPCS	Office of Population Censuses and Surveys
PA	Plasminogen activator
PALA	*N*-(phosphonacetyl)-L-aspartate
RFLP	Restriction fragment length polymorphism
SD	Sprague Dawley
SDF	Soluble dietary fibres
TGF-β	Transforming growth factor-beta
TPA	12-*O*-tetradecanoylphorbol-13-acetate

1

Development of the disease

Colorectal cancer is of particular interest to the cancer scientist, because it is the one cancer that presents as a consequence of the progression of the normal tissue through a histologically identifiable pre-malignant state to frank malignancy. Colorectal cancer therefore has a clear multistage and possibly multifactorial aetiology which is consistent with some of the best models and theories of carcinogenesis. However, no scientific study can be conducted in ignorance of the clinical background to the disease and the diversity of factors that influence both the acquisition of malignancy and its prognosis. In countries like the United States and the United Kingdom where diets are high in fats and cholesterol and low in fibre, colorectal cancer continues to be one of the most frequently encountered tumours in both men and women. It is the second commonest cancer in the United Kingdom with approximately 17 000 people dying from it annually.

The polyp–cancer sequence

There are a large variety of tumour types that involve the large bowel, but the overwhelming majority of large bowel tumours are adenocarcinomas, which have arisen from pre-existing benign adenomatous polyps or villous adenomas in what is known as the polyp–cancer sequence (Grinell and Lane, 1958; Welch, 1964; Morson, 1965; Hill, 1975). Adenomas may occur singly or in their thousands in patients with familial polyposis coli (FPC) or what is now commonly called familial adenomatous polyposis (FAP). The term adenoma encompasses sessile, semi-sessile and pedunculated polypoid growths, which histologically can be divided into three types: (1) tubular adenomas, consisting of proliferating tubules, (2) villous adenomas, composed of finger-like fronds clothed in atypical epithelia and (3) intermediate tubulo-villous adenomas (Fig. 1.1).

Tubular adenomas account for 75 per cent of adenomas, the typical villous adenoma for 10 per cent and the tubulo-villous adenomas for about 15 per cent. However, the malignancy rate is only 5 per cent for the common tubular adenoma compared with 40 per cent for villous adenomas and 22 per cent for the intermediate tubulo-villous adenoma (Morson, 1974). So, how are these discrepancies in malignant potential explained?

The incidence of cancer in polyps is broadly related to polyp size, histological type and degree of differentiation. The risk of malignant change is only about 1 per cent in adenomas up to 1 cm in size. The proportion rises to 10 per cent in those 1–2 cm in size and 38–50 per cent in those over 2 cm in size (Morson, 1974; Gillespie *et al.*, 1979). The common tubular adenoma is usually small and therefore, as might be predicted, rarely contains invasive cancer (Muto *et al.*, 1975). Typically the villous adenoma presents as a larger tumour and even the small ones of these have a malignancy rate approaching 10 per cent which rises to greater than 50 per cent in tumours more than 2 cm in size. Cancer incidence also increases with epithelial dysplasia. The criteria for judging the degree of epithelial dysplasia include nuclear changes, pleomorphism, loss of polar-

Fig. 1.1. Adenomas of large intestinal mucosa: variations in structure (Talbot, 1982).

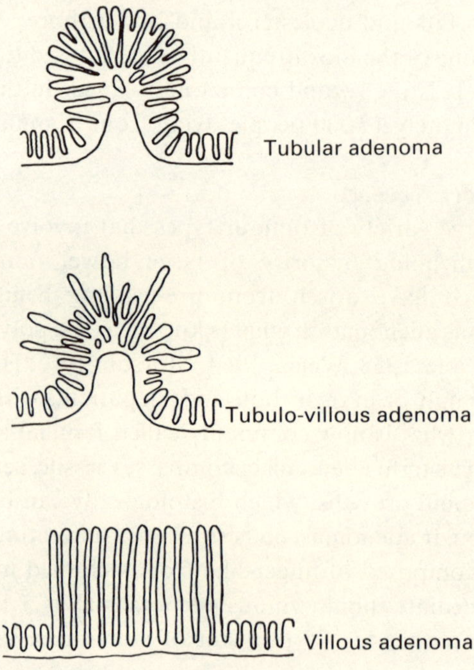

ity, stratification and an increase in the number of mitotic figures. Data from St Mark's Hospital, London (Muto *et al.*, 1975), show that small polyps very rarely show severe dysplasia, but that when they do, there is a high malignant potential. As polyps get larger the influence of the degree of dysplasia on malignant potential diminishes. Therefore, size is of great importance when trying to assess malignant potential. The malignancy rate for all tubular adenomas with mild or moderate dysplasia, which are the great majority, is low. Severe dysplasia in tubular adenomas is rare, but when it occurs it is associated with high malignant potential. In contrast, villous adenomas often show severe dysplasia which again is consistent with an increased malignant potential. Overall, 5–20 per cent of polyps are found to contain either invasive carcinoma or carcinoma *in situ*.

It is not known how long it takes for an adenoma to become malignant and early tumours normally retain the configuration of the pre-existing adenoma before eventually becoming fungating growths. A single adenoma observed at the Mayo Clinic only developed malignant change after 15 years (Mayo and de Castro, 1956) whilst three out of four solitary, untreated tubular adenomas studied at St Mark's in London, developed their malignant changes after 5, 6 and 13 years, respectively (Morson, 1976). Life history studies of ten villous adenomas were made over periods ranging from 5 to 30 years. During this time in spite of numerous benign tumour recurrences only two progressed to carcinoma after 10 and 28 years respectively, suggesting that the villous adenoma–carcinoma sequence is probably not inevitable (Morson, 1976). However, age distribution curves for benign and malignant tumours of the colon and rectum (Fig. 1.2) show that single tubular and villous adenomas are recognised on average 4 years before carcinomas, at 58.1 and 62.1 years respectively.

This, however, is likely to be a gross underestimate because tubular adenomas and villous adenomas are often symptomless and are discovered as a consequence of some other condition of the bowel. Therefore all the evidence discussed so far suggests that the time course of the adenoma–carcinoma sequence must be at least 5 years. A further insight into the time course for malignant change comes from a study at St Mark's of 3002 patients who already had malignant disease (Morson, 1974). Of these 2412 had only one tumour, whilst 590 (19.7 per cent) had multiple single tumours that were either benign or malignant. Thus, 1 in 5 patients with neoplastic disease of the large bowel have more than one benign or malignant lesion elsewhere in the colon or rectum. In the same series of 3002 patients, 210 (7 per cent) developed a second metachronous benign or malignant tumour that was detected during routine follow-up examination. The interval between the first and second cancers in this particular study varied from 2 to 31 years with the average being 13.5 years. The life history of the polyp–cancer sequence as exemplified by this study is very variable. The risk varies depending on whether or not tubular or villous adenomas are present in the first operation specimen, but it does demonstrate that the polyp–cancer sequence is a process that evolves over a period of years.

Nowhere is this better demonstrated than in familial polyposis coli (FPC), also known as familial adenomatous polyposis (FAP), a genetically predetermined condition in which the mucous membrane of the large intestine is carpeted by hundreds or thousands of polyps. Most of these are tubular adenomas although a minority are villous and intermediate adenomas. This is pertinent to our theories of the time scale for the development of cancer from isolated tubular adenomas and villous adenomas, because these patients if left untreated will inevitably get cancer. Age distribution curves for polyposis and cancer (Fig. 1.3) show that the average age at diagnosis of polyposis without cancer is 27 years and of polyposis with cancer is 39 years (Morson, 1974). This gives a time interval of about 12 years between the diagnosis of polyposis and the development of cancer; this is likely to be an underestimate because polyposis in the early stages is likely to be asymptomatic.

Further information on this subject comes from the analysis of the age of onset of polyposis and cancer in patients who did not have any treatment for their disease. Of 59 patients with polyposis only 7 developed

Fig. 1.2. Age distribution for benign and malignant tumours of the colon and rectum (Morson, 1976).

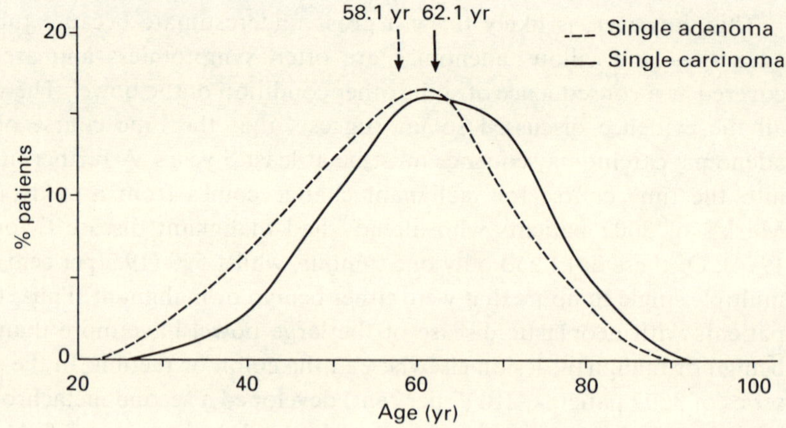

cancer during the first 5 years, a further 10 during the next 5 years, and by 15–20 years 50 per cent of patients had developed cancer with only 4 patients having polyposis that remained benign for 20 years. Thus, these data lend support to the notion that the evolution of cancer of the colon and rectum takes at least 5 years and can take more than 20 years, but on average takes between 15 and 20 years. However, studies have not only been made of the development of the malignancy, but also of the doubling times of tumour volume once the malignant change has taken place. Direct measurements of tumour growth in 20 patients by Welin *et al.* (1963) showed a mean doubling time of 620 days. Studies by Charbit *et al.* (1971), however, showed primary tumours to have a tumour volume doubling time of only 207 days. In the same study, a metastatic adenocarcinoma had a doubling time of 90 days. An awareness of the variability in the development of the disease, and of the aggressiveness of the disease once it has developed, is essential for a proper scientific evaluation of any scientific observations made.

Mode of presentation and pathology

The determinants which affect prognosis include the size of the tumour. As suggested above, smaller tumours carry a better prognosis. The presence of an obstruction halves the number of patients surviving compared with those with a non-obstructing lesion. Also, patients with carcinomas of the right side of the colon have a poorer prognosis quite simply because their carcinomas are quite advanced before they produce

Fig. 1.3. Age distribution for polyposis and cancer (Morson, 1976).

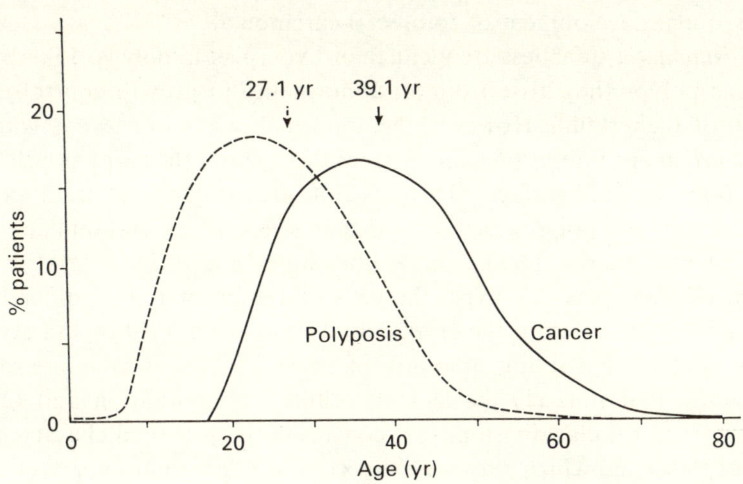

any symptoms. However, possibly the single most important determinant of prognosis is the degree of spread at the time of surgical treatment.

The wall of the colon and rectum is composed of several discrete layers that include the mucosa, the submucosa, the muscularis propria and the serosa. Strictly speaking a polyp is any bump or protrusion of the mucosal surface. This bump may be the result of a proliferation of the mucosal surface itself or it may be the consequence of the proliferation of structures lying deep to the mucosa, i.e. structures in the submucosa, muscularis propria, etc. Non-mucosal polypoid proliferations give rise to lesions such as lipomas, leiomyomas and lymphoid polyps and can be distinguished both grossly and endoscopically from epithelial mucosal polyps. However, it is only the epithelial mucosal polyps in which we are interested, in terms of colorectal carcinoma, of which polyps or adenomas are only one subset.

Classification of epithelial mucosal polyps

Hyperplastic polyps result from an abnormality in cell division within the crypt of Lieberkühn in which the replicating zone is expanded (Kaye *et al.*, 1973, Fenoglio *et al.*, 1977). This results in the presence of actively dividing cells in the lower half of the crypt. The increased mitotic activity gives rise to a larger than normal number of cells which in turn results in the formation of small mucosal polyps with distinctive serrated lumens. Interestingly, although cell division is increased, there is eventual differentiation into mature adult intestinal cells. It is this eventual cessation of cell division and subsequent differentiation that distinguishes the non-neoplastic hyperplastic polyp from the neoplastic adenomatous polyp. Purely hyperplastic polyps have no apparent relationship to the subsequent development of colorectal carcinoma.

Adenomas are far less frequent than hyperplastic polyps. Like hyperplastic polyps they arise from an abnormality in growth control in the crypt of Lieberkühn. However, the abnormality is more severe, with cell division and proliferation being present throughout the crypt as well as on the free luminal surface. This loss of growth control leads to the production of a polyp which can range in size from several millimetres to several centimetres. Unlike the epithelium of the normal crypt, or the crypt of hyperplastic polyps, the cells of the crypt fail to differentiate completely. As a result, the crypts of adenomas are lined by tall atypical cells containing varying amounts of mucin. Thus, it is important to recognise that it is (1) the lack of cellular differentiation and (2) the unrestricted cellular division, that constitute the principal characteristics of neoplasia and which allow one to recognise adenomatous epithelium as being neoplastic and a precursor for the subsequent development of colorectal carcinoma.

Adenomatous polyps with hyperplastic features are difficult to categorise as either hyperplastic or adenomatous.

Juvenile polyps are generally pedunculated non-neoplastic growths composed of cystically dilated glands. The stalks of juvenile polyps are lined by normal mucosa. These lesions are typically solitary and usually occur in the rectum or sigmoid colon.

Peutz–Jeghers polyps are pedunculated, hamartomatous, non-neoplastic lesions that range in size from 0.1 to 3 cm. They are composed of mature non-dividing intestinal epithelial cells.

Generally speaking, however, there is a continuum of neoplastic change that occurs in the colon and rectum which is difficult to compartmentalise in any way, but which starts with the formation of a neoplastic but benign adenomatous gland. The next step is the presence of cells that are cytologically malignant, yet are confined to the original contours of the crypt of Lieberkühn without invasion of the neighbouring lamina propria. The next step is invasion into the lamina propria by malignant-looking glands without extension through the muscularis mucosae, and finally the presence of invasive carcinoma which invades the muscularis mucosae. There is little doubt that the survival of patients with colorectal cancer is inversely proportional to the extent of local invasion, with a marked decrease being apparent once the tumour has penetrated the muscularis mucosae. In an attempt to 'stage' colorectal carcinoma Dukes in 1936 introduced what became known as the Dukes' classification, and although some clinicians have thought to modify it slightly (Kirklin *et al.*, 1949; Astler and Coller, 1954), it is still employed essentially in its original form, which is as follows:

Stage A. Tumours limited to the bowel wall with no extension through the serosa.

Stage B. Tumours which have penetrated the muscularis propria by direct continuity, but have not invaded the lymph nodes.

Stage C. Tumours which have penetrated all layers of the bowel wall, with metastases present in the regional nodes.

However, in addition to lymphatic spread colorectal carcinomas can be considered to have three modes of spread: (1) The tumour may spread for short distances into the submucosa and muscle tissues and may spread laterally to adjacent structures (Williams *et al.*, 1983). The extent of this local invasion is a major determinant of survival. (2) The second important pattern of spread is via venous invasion, which frequently results in the development of liver metastases. Thirty to fifty per cent of cases can have liver involvement (Finlay *et al.*, 1982). (3) The third mode of spread is via the trans-coelomic route to produce carcinomatosis peritonei.

Thus, to summarise so far, the 5-year survival can be between 70 and 90 per cent in asymptomatic patients, whilst the duration of the symptoms has little bearing on the prognosis, because short symptom duration normally correlates with more aggressive disease. Finally patients under 30 years of age were thought to have a very poor prognosis, whilst survival in the elderly was thought to be greater because their malignancy was of a lower pathological grade (Dukes and Bussey, 1958). However, modern data suggest that the prognosis gets worse with increasing age.

Individuals at risk of developing colorectal carcinoma

Persons at the highest risk of developing colorectal carcinoma and who will do so in 100 per cent of cases unless they undergo total colectomy, are patients with FPC (FAP). As stated previously the bowel wall in these patients is carpeted with hundreds or thousands of tubular polyps. These polyps occur in young patients and can give rise to numerous synchronous or metachronous carcinomas at a younger age than in the normal population (Bussey, 1975; Decosse *et al.*, 1977; Lynch and Krush, 1967; Lynch *et al.*, 1979). Other polyposis syndromes include Gardner's syndrome (Gardner, 1951) and Turcot's syndrome, both of which involve large numbers of adenomatous polyps and an increased incidence of colorectal cancer (Erbe, 1976; Lynch *et al.*, 1979). In the latter two disorders, in addition to the intestinal polyposis, the patients manifest a variety of extra-intestinal changes, which will be detailed in the following chapter. There are also polyposis syndromes which involve proliferations of juvenile polyps (Goodman *et al.*, 1979; Stemper *et al.*, 1975; Haggitt and Pitcock, 1970). These patients have an increased risk of developing colorectal cancer as do members of their family, but it does not approach that of Gardner's syndrome or Turcot's syndrome. Similarly there is an increased risk of developing cancer in patients with Peutz–Jeghers syndrome in whom hamartomatous polyps are present (Rozen and Baratz, 1982). Other individuals at increased risk of developing colorectal cancer are those who already have adenomatous polyps. The risk increases with increasing numbers of polyps, particularly in those patients who are members of the so-called colon cancer families. The younger the patient when cancer develops and the presence of multiple adenomas in the resected specimen the greater the risk that a subsequent cancer will develop (Heald and Lockhart-Mummery, 1972). Analysis of family histories of patients undergoing treatment for colorectal cancer has shown the number of deaths from colorectal cancer in first degree relatives to be approximately three times that observed in a comparable normal group (Lovett, 1976). Patients with inflammatory bowel disease are also known to be at increased risk of developing large bowel cancer (Ridell *et al.*, 1983). Ulcerative colitis is associated with a 5- to 10-fold increased risk of colorectal carcinoma, the risk being dependent upon the extent of the disease and the length of the history. Cancer generally only develops in patients where colitis involves most of the large intestine (Lennard-Jones *et al.*, 1977).

References

Astler, V. B. and Coller, F. A. (1954) The prognostic significance of direct extension of carcinoma of the colon and rectum. *Ann. Surg.*, **139**, 846.

Bussey, H. J. R. (1975) *Familial Polyposis Coli.* Johns Hopkins University Press, Baltimore.

Charbit, A., Malaise, E. P. and Tubiana, M. (1971) Relation between pathological nature and growth of human tumours. *Eur. J. Cancer*, **7**, 307.

DeCosse, J. J., Adams, M. B. and Condon, R. E. (1977) Familial polyposis coli. *Cancer*, **39**, 267–73.

Dukes, C. E. (1936) Histological grading of rectal cancer. *Proc. R. Soc. Med.*, **30**, 371–6.

Dukes, C. E. and Bussey, H. J. R. (1958) The spread of rectal cancer and its effect on prognosis. *Br. J. Cancer*, **12**, 309–20.

Erbe, R. W. (1976) Inherited gastrointestinal-polyposis syndromes. *New Engl. J. Med.*, **294**, 1101–4.

Fenoglio, C. M., Kaye, G. I., Pascal, P. R. and Lane, N. (1977) Defining the precursor tissue of ordinary large bowel carcinoma: implications for cancer prevention. *Pathol. Annu.*, **12**, 87.

Finlay, I. G., Meek, D. R., Gray, H. W., Duncan, J. G. and McCardle, C. S. (1982) Incidence and detection of occult hepatic metastases in colorectal carcinoma. *Br. Med. J.*, **284**, 803–5.

Gardner, E. J. (1951) A genetic and clinical study of intestinal polyposis, a predisposing factor for carcinoma of the colon and rectum. *Am. J. Hum. Genet.*, **3**, 167–76.

Gillespie, P. E., Chambers, T. J., Chan, K., *et al.* (1979) Colonic adenomas: a colonoscopy survey. *Gut*, **20**, 240–5.

Goodman, Z. D., Yardley, J. H. and Milligan, F. D. (1979) Pathogenesis of colonic polyps in multiple juvenile polyposis. *Cancer*, **43**, 1906–13.

Grinell, R. S. and Lane, N. (1958) Benign and malignant adenomatous polyps and papillary adenomas of the colon and rectum: an analysis of 1856 tumours in 1335 patients. *Surgery*, **106**, 519–38.

Haggitt, R. C. and Pitcock, J. A. (1970) Familial juvenile polyposis of the colon. *Cancer*, **26**, 1232–8.

Heald, R. J. and Lockhart-Mummery, H. E. (1972) The lesion of the second cancer of the large bowel. *Br. J. Surg.*, **59**, 16.

Hill, M. J. (1975) The role of colonic anaerobes in the metabolism of bile acids and steroids and its relation to colon cancer. *Cancer*, **36**, 2387–400.

Kaye, G. I., Fenoglio, C. M., Pascal, R. R. and Lane, N. (1973) Comparative electron microscopic features of normal, hyperplastic and adenomatous human colonic epithelium: variations in cellular structure relative to the process of epithelial differentiation. *Gastroenterology*, **64**, 926.

Kirklin, J. W., Dockerty, M. B. and Waugh, J. M. (1949) The role of the peritoneal reflection in the prognosis of carcinoma of the rectum and the sigmoid colon. *Surg. Gynecol. Obstet.*, **88**, 326–31.

Lennard-Jones, J. E., Morson, B. C., Ritchie, J. K., Shove, D. C. and Williams, C. B. (1977) Cancer in colitis: assessment of the individual risk by clinical and histological criteria. *Gastroenterology*, **73**, 1280–9.

Lovett, E. (1976) Family studies in cancer of the colon and rectum. *Por. J. Surg.*, **63**, 13–18.

Lynch, H. T. and Krush, A. J. (1967) Heredity and adenocarcinoma of the colon. *Gastroenterology*, **53**, 517–27.

Lynch, H. T., Lynch, P. M., Follett, K. L. and Harris, R. E. (1979) Familial polyposis coli: heterogeneous polyp expression in 2 kindreds. *J. Med. Genet.*, **16**, 1–7.

Mayo, C. W. and de Castro, C. A. (1956) Carcinoma of the sigmoid arising from a polyp first visualised 15 years previously: report of a case. *Proc. Mayo Clin.*, **31**, 597–8

Morson, B. C. (1965) Notes on the pathology of carcinoma of the large intestine. *Natl. Cancer Inst. Monogr.*, **25**.

Morson, B. C. (1974) The polyp–cancer sequence in the large bowel. *Proc. R. Soc. Med.*, **67**, 451–7.

Morson, B. C. (1976) Genesis of colorectal cancer. *Clin. Gastroenterol.*, **3**, 505–25.

Muto, T., Bussey, H. J. R. and Morson, B. C. (1975) The evolution of cancer of the colon and rectum. *Cancer*, **36**, 2251–70.

Ridell, R. H., Goldman, H., Ransohoff, D. F., *et al.* (1983) Dysplasia in inflammatory bowel disease: standardised classification with provisional clinical applications. *Hum. Pathol.*, **14**, 931–68.

Rozen, P. and Baratz, M. (1982) Familial juvenile colonic polyposis with associated colon cancer. *Cancer*, **49**, 1500–3.

Stemper, T. J., Kent, T. H. and Summers, R. W. (1975) Juvenile polyposis and gastrointestinal carcinoma. *Ann. Intern. Med.*, **83**, 639–46.

Talbot, I. C. (1982) Pathology and natural history. In: *Colorectal Cancer*, ed. W. Duncan, pp. 59–66. Springer, Berlin.

Welch, C. E. (1964) *Polypoid Lesions of the Gastrointestinal Tract*. Saunders, Philadelphia.

Welin, J., Youker, J. and Spratt, J. S. (1963) The rates and patterns of 375 tumours of the large intestine and rectum observed serially by double contrast enema study (Malmo technique). *Am. J. Roentgenol.*, **90**, 673–87.

Williams, N. S., Dixon, M. F. and Johnston, D. (1983) Re-appraisal of the 5-cm rule of distal excision for carcinoma of the rectum: a study of distal intramural spread and patient survival. *Por. J. Surg.*, **70**, 150–4.

2

Conditions associated with increased susceptibility

Genetically linked polyposis syndromes

In man, the role of hereditary factors in the aetiology of most malignant neoplasms is uncertain. However, several disorders of the colon such as FPC (FAP), Gardner's syndrome, Peutz–Jeghers syndrome, juvenile polyposis and Turcot's syndrome, which all predispose in varying degrees to malignancy, exhibit a strong genetic basis.

Familial polyposis coli

Familial polyposis coli (FPC), also commonly known as familial adenomatous polyposis (FAP), was first described by Cripps in 1882. It has a classical autosomal dominant mode of inheritance, with the gene provisionally assigned to chromosome 5 (Bodmer *et al.*, 1987). The incidence of FPC has been reported by a variety of authors to be anything between 1 in 6850 and 1 in 23 950 live births (Neel, 1954; Veale, 1965; Pierce, 1968; Bussey, 1975; Erbe, 1976), with a penetrance estimated to be 90 per cent (Reed and Neel, 1955). About 20 per cent of patients appear to be the first in their families to be affected, a pattern totally consistent with a fresh autosomal dominant mutation being the cause of their disease. However, some of these cases may only appear to be sporadic because of a failure to detect the disease in relatives.

The disease is characterised by the occurrence of numerous, predominantly tubular adenomas or polyps, which commonly carpet the entire colon and rectum. Some of these adenomas have a villous component and can be classified as tubulo-villous, but a pure villous adenoma is, according to Morson (1976), exceptional in an FPC patient. The polyp number can vary between a few hundred to a few thousand, but commonly averages around a thousand (Erbe, 1976). No case of true FPC has ever been reported in relatives of patients with less than 100 polyps

(Bussey, 1975), although marked variability in the frequency and location of polyps has been reported in two extended American kindreds supposedly manifesting FPC (Lynch *et al.*, 1979). The predisposition to carcinoma, as described in the preceding chapter (Chapter 1), is striking. The observed incidence of neoplasms in untreated patients is approximately 80 per cent and it seems likely, therefore, that all patients would develop carcinoma if left untreated. The natural course of polyposis can be summarised as follows from data obtained from 207 polyposis patients for whom little was known other than that they died of intestinal cancer (Bussey, 1975):

Age at appearance of adenomas	24.5 years
Age at onset of symptoms	33.0 years
Age at diagnosis of adenomas	35.8 years
Age at diagnosis of carcinoma	39.2 years
Age at death from cancer	42.0 years

This group was chosen to assess the age distribution at death because it consisted mainly of an older generation who belonged to a time when surgery was both less frequent and less effective. There is little difference between the sexes in incidence and in the age at diagnosis (Fig. 2.1),

Fig. 2.1. Age distribution at the time of diagnosis of males and females with polyposis for 281 propositus cases (Bussey, 1975).

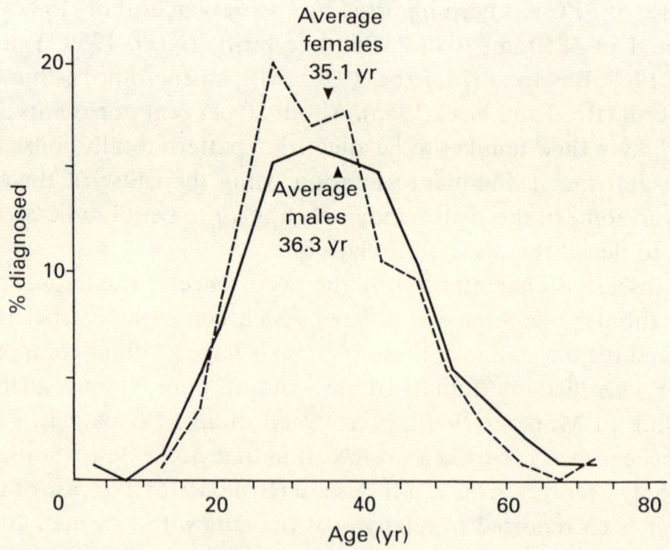

as assessed from 281 polyposis patients who presented because they had symptoms (Bussey, 1975). The same group provided useful information about the proportion of cases diagnosed at increasing age (Fig. 2.2).

Interestingly, although FPC is considered to be a disease of young adults or at worst early middle age, these data show that by 35 years of age only half the cases have been diagnosed. The data also demonstrate the risk at various ages of still developing malignancy for the apparently unaffected offspring of a polyposis patient. It should be remembered, therefore, that the age of onset can be very variable and can range from 4 months to 74 years (Stauffer, 1973). At the time of diagnosis, at an average age of 39 years, two-thirds of the probands (the first members of their families to be diagnosed) already have a carcinoma and multiple primary lesions are to be found at operation. Hence, adenocarcinoma in these patients develops approximately 20 years earlier than in patients without polyposis (Morson, 1976; Fig. 1.2) and multiple primary tumours are about 12 times more frequent (Bussey *et al.*, 1967). In fact, FPC provides a valuable model of malignancy where a germ cell mutation and presumably environmental factors (mutagens) combine to accelerate the normal progression of the disease. Detailed studies of the tissues and cells of such patients should provide an insight into more common neoplasias, particularly as there is evidence that some of the benign lesions of the colon are reversible (Cole and Holden, 1959; Cole *et al.*, 1961).

Fig. 2.2. The percentage of 281 polyposis cases diagnosed at different ages. At 35 years of age half the cases have been diagnosed whilst at 50 years there are still more than 10 per cent of the propositus patients who have not presented (Bussey, 1975).

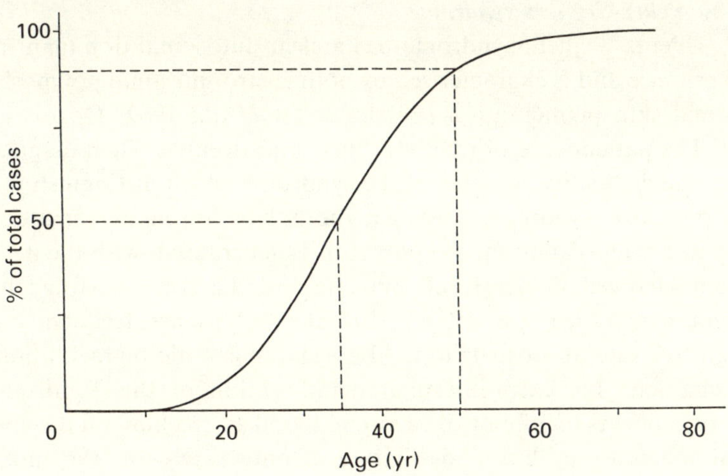

Gardner's syndrome

Gardner's syndrome (GS) is another of the classical polyposis syndromes, but in addition to intestinal polyposis, patients can have soft tissue abnormalities and bone abnormalities (Gardner, 1951, 1962). It is, however, unusual for patients to manifest all three types of abnormality and generally it is only through the study of several family members that this syndrome can be distinguished from FPC. The polyps are normally found in the colon and rectum although a few cases of polyps in the small intestine and stomach have been reported. They are histologically indistinguishable from those of FPC patients and their mean age of onset, diagnosis and liability to progress to adenocarcinoma are essentially identical. The principal differences between FPC and GS were thought to be the higher number of polyps in FPC, defined by Bussey (1975) as greater than 100, and the lack of extracolonic expression in FPC. It was commonly thought that in GS the polyps were more scattered and the mucosa less carpeted (Bussey, 1975). Thus, FPC and GS were considered to be separate genotypes with the common features of autosomal dominant inheritance and adenomatous colonic polyps. However, we are now aware that certain extracolonic lesions, such as gastric and duodenal polyps, occur in at least 68 per cent of patients with FPC. These findings, along with the increased incidence of periampullary malignancy in both FPC and GS, suggest that these diseases are not separate genotypes but represent the varying expressivity of a single, pleotropic gene (Smith, 1958, 1968; Harned and Williams, 1982). For the purpose of this book, therefore, patients with FPC and GS will be assumed to have the same propensity for colonic malignancy.

Peutz–Jeghers syndrome

Peutz–Jeghers syndrome has a clear autosomal dominant mode of inheritance and is characterised by both gastro-intestinal polyposis and abnormal skin pigmentation (Bartholomew *et al.*, 1962; Dozois *et al.*, 1969). The patients are normally in their mid-twenties when diagnosis is made. The distinctive features of the syndrome which distinguish it from other polyposis syndromes are that the polyps are hamartomatous (of embryonic origin) and that the polyposis is generalised, with the ileum or jejunum involved in nearly all patients and the rectum, stomach and duodenum involved less often. Also, the polyps are frequently large enough to cause an obstruction. Abnormal melanotic pigmentation is a very characteristic extra-intestinal manifestation of this syndrome. It normally appears in infancy or early childhood as 'freckles' on the lips and buccal mucosae, eyelids and digits and only rarely on the intestinal mucosae. The pigmentation on the lips is the most consistent, but tends to fade with age and also unfortunately is not uncommon in individuals who do not have this syndrome. However, it is now recognised that those individuals with the syndrome have a 2–3 per cent risk of gastro-intestinal carcinoma, often involving the duodenal region (Dozois *et al.*, 1969; Case Records Massachussetts General Hospital, 1975).

Juvenile polyposis

Juvenile polyposis is a rare syndrome with an autosomal dominant mode of inheritance with complete penetrance and is normally but not exclusively diagnosed in the first decade of life (Veale *et al.*, 1966; Smilow *et al.*, 1966; Sachatello *et al.*, 1974; Gathright and Cofer, 1974). In some cases it is thought to be congenital. It nearly always involves the colon and rectum although rarely the small intestine and stomach. Juvenile polyps of the colon are usually solitary lesions (Goodman *et al.*, 1979) and are clearly inflammatory lesions or hamartomas which have become secondarily inflamed (Morson, 1962; Roth and Helwig, 1963). Seventy per cent of patients have single polyps and the remainder have two or three and only very rarely as many as ten (Haggitt and Pitcock, 1970). There are no extra-intestinal manifestations of the disease as in Gardner's and Peutz–Jeghers syndromes.

Recently it has been observed that the polyps of some of these patients may show epithelial atypia and may take on a distinctly adenomatous appearance. The possibility was therefore raised that the presence of epithelial atypia may represent a pre-malignant lesion in some of these cases (Goodman *et al.*, 1979). For example, a patient with a non-familial case of multiple juvenile polyposis in which there were five categories of lesions developed a rectal carcinoma aged 23 years (Goodman *et al.*, 1979). Smilow *et al.* (1966) reported three cases of juvenile polyposis in three generations of one family. The oldest patient also had colon carcinoma. Haggitt and Pitcock (1970) reported two cases of juvenile polyposis in two generations of a family with a high incidence of colonic carcinoma. Stemper *et al.* (1975) described a kindred in which at least 10 members had single or multiple juvenile polyps of the stomach and large intestine and 11 members had gastro-intestinal cancer. However, in the particular kindred studied by Stemper *et al.* (1975) the carcinomas described were not related closely to the polyps either in location or time of appearance, raising the possibility that the neoplasms result from the action of the gene rather than being secondary to the polyposis (Erbe, 1976). More recently, Rozen and Baratz (1982) reported multiple juvenile polyposis of the colon in a mother and son in a family where no other known family member had shown evidence of a polyposis syndrome or had a history of malignancy. Later the mother developed a metastatic adenocarcinoma of the colon. In both patients the juvenile polyps contained adenomatous features. Again, it was postulated that juvenile polyps may undergo dysplasia in middle life leading to an increased risk of malignancy (Rozen and Baratz, 1982 and refs. therein) and that adenomatous-style dysplasia could be a marker of potential malignancy in these patients.

Turcot's syndrome

Turcot's syndrome is the least well established of the polyposis syndromes, having been described thoroughly in only two families (Turcot *et al.*, 1959; Baughman *et al.*, 1969), although other isolated cases have been reported (Crail, 1949; Camiel *et al.*, 1968; Bussey, 1975). As seen above the differences between the other polyposis syndromes are in the nature and location of the polyps and in the extra-intestinal lesions. Turcot's syndrome is characterised by the presence of adenomatous polyps and a distinctive inheritance pattern. In two healthy families, two healthy parents had two and four children respectively with polyposis and some form of brain tumour, suggesting that there is an autosomal recessive pattern of inheritance (Turcot *et al.*, 1959; Baughman *et al.* 1969). These cases could be interpreted as showing a predisposition to some form of brain tumour rather than a tumour of the gastro-intestinal tract, although this might quite simply reflect a difference in the time course for development – because, after all, the polyposis is already present. It is also postulated that Turcot's syndrome might be another manifestation of the unusual tumours found in Gardner's syndrome.

Family history

Cancer of the large bowel other than that associated with the polyposis syndromes has not until recently been considered a familial disease, although adenocarcinoma of the colon in the absence of polyps has been shown to occur frequently in certain families (Lynch and Krush, 1967; Lovett, 1976). First degree relatives of patients with 'sporadic' colorectal carcinoma have a 2- to 3-fold increased risk of the same cancer (Lovett, 1976) and several studies have reported an increased prevalence of adenomatous polyps among relatives of patients with colorectal carcinoma. It is now estimated that 5 per cent or more of the patients with colorectal carcinoma inherit their disease as an autosomal dominant trait (Mulvihill, 1983; Lynch and Lynch 1985). Lynch *et al.* (1985) defined these clearly familial cases as Lynch syndrome I for familial site-specific, non-polyposis colon cancer and Lynch syndrome II (CFS, cancer family syndrome) for familial site-specific, non-polyposis colon cancer associated with other forms of cancer. These two subgroups were subsequently named hereditary non-polyposis colorectal cancer (HNPCC) types a and b. However, because much of the evidence predates these later definitions, all definitions will be included in the sub-headings below.

Colon cancer families (Lynch syndrome I, HNPCC type a)

Several reports have appeared of families in which there is a high incidence of carcinoma of the large bowel. Woolf *et al.* (1955) described a family in which there was a high incidence of adenocarcinoma in one generation. Screening of 55 members of the next generation showed 25 of these individuals to have one or more polyps. Woolf *et al.* (1955) suggested that such a family aggregation could be due to the inheritance of discrete or solitary polyps and that if this was the case then close relatives should also have an increased incidence of large bowel cancer (Woolf, 1958). That close relatives did indeed have an increased incidence of the disease was confirmed by examining the deaths from large bowel cancer in the State of Utah using the Mormon genealogical records.

Macklin (1960) studied the family histories of 145 patients who had had surgery for large bowel cancer in hospitals in one city in the USA. Although follow-up showed an increased incidence of intestinal cancer among first and second degree relatives, she could not find any simple pattern of inheritance to account for the increased incidence.

Dunstone and Knaggs (1972) described a family in which 22 out of 50 recorded deaths were due to carcinoma of the colon or rectum. In addition, five surviving members of the family had had carcinoma of the large bowel diagnosed and treated. The affected individuals were members of three generations and in only one family member was a benign polyp diagnosed and treated, eliminating any possibility that a polyposis syndrome was responsible for the high incidence.

Lovett (1976) investigated the records of 209 patients with carcinoma of the large bowel admitted to St Mark's Hospital in London for an increased incidence of the disease amongst first degree relatives and again confirmed that close relatives of patients with large bowel cancer are themselves more likely to develop large bowel cancer than members of the general population.

The affected individuals in such colon cancer families also tended to develop cancer at an earlier age than would be expected in the normal population (Woolf *et al.*, 1955; Macklin, 1960; Lovett, 1976), but in none of the cases could a familial polyposis syndrome be considered responsible. Also, it was considered at this time unlikely that a simple, single locus hereditary factor was involved and thought that more complex genetic mechanisms and diet might play an important role.

More recently, however, investigation of the inherited susceptibility to colonic polyps and carcinomas in a large Utah pedigree (Burt *et al.*, 1985) has suggested that the observed increased incidence within certain families was consistent with an inherited autosomal dominant trait. This type of inheritance of colorectal polyps might be more common than previously recognised. In a study by Bonelli *et al.* (1988) family history was associated with a similarly increased risk of both adenomatous polyps and carcinoma. This supports the hypothesis that a single locus genetic factor is involved in the familial clustering of 'sporadic' colon carcinomas and that it is involved in the early stages of the multi-step progression to colon carcinogenesis by increasing the risk of adenomatous polyps. However, environmental factors must be considered as possible causative agents where familial groups are concerned, as the individuals concerned are very likely to have been exposed to the same environmental agents. Therefore, in colon cancer families one can speculate that hereditary factors are present which interact with common environmental factors such as diet to produce an increased risk of cancer.

Cancer family syndrome (Lynch syndrome II, HNPCC type b)

The study of 'cancer families' which were characterised by a high occurrence of cancers at different anatomical sites, uncovered a further hereditary aetiology for carcinoma of the colon together with carcinoma of the endometrium (Warthin, 1913, 1925; Mathis, 1962; Kluge, 1964). Lynch and Krush (1967), in a study of six cancer families, revealed an exceedingly high incidence of cancer, particularly cancer of the colon, but in the complete absence once again of a polyposis syndrome. For example, in family 1, of thirteen siblings seven showed carcinoma. Four of these had multiple carcinomas, of which colon carcinoma was one in each case. In family 2, colon carcinoma appeared in three generations. In family 3, adenocarcinoma of the colon appeared in four generations. Colon carcinoma appeared in five generations in family 5 (Warthin's family G) and of ten individuals with multiple primary malignancies, eight had carcinomas of the colon. In family 6, eleven members in three generations had malignant neoplasms all of which involved the colon. Analysis of the pedigrees of these families, and others (Savage, 1956; Heizelmann, 1964; Lynch and Lynch, 1987), showed adenocarcinoma of the colon to be transmitted in a pattern consistent with an autosomal dominant mode of inheritance, with an increased occurrence of multiple primary malignancies associated with colon carcinoma and an early age of onset. In these families the proximal colon is affected in 65 per cent of cases whilst 65–80 per cent of sporadic colon carcinomas and those associated with FPC (FAP) are associated with the distal colon (Lynch *et al.*, 1977).

Recently, the frequency of hereditary colorectal carcinoma was evaluated in a study group consisting of all the colorectal carcinoma patients diagnosed between 1970 and 1979 in one county of Finland (Mecklin, 1987). The 'cancer family syndrome' type of non-polyposis colorectal carcinoma emerged as the most common verifiable risk factor for colon carcinoma (Mecklin, 1987). In family screening of HNPCC individuals, positive screening results were at least 20–30 times higher than in the same age group in the general population (Mecklin, 1989). Thus, it seems that inherited susceptibility constitutes a very significant risk factor. The site-specific presentation of colorectal carcinoma has been reported in two pairs of identical twins. In one pair, with a family history, the presentation was simultaneous, at 57 years of age (Winkler *et al.*, 1983). The other pair presented 2 years apart, at 32 and 34 years of age, with no family history (Whitehead, 1980). In another instance, identical twins presented within 5 months of each other with multiple primary colonic tumours (Johnson and Thomson, 1986). Although the data indicate that in the majority of cases of colorectal carcinoma in monozygotic twins only one twin is affected (Jarvik and Falek, 1962; Lovett, 1976), in the three reports cited above the twins shared genetic as well as environmental factors which might have been relevant to the development of the disease. These reports may therefore represent extreme examples of a familial predisposition to the non-polyposis form of the disease.

Previous history of carcinoma or adenoma

Individuals who have had cancer removed from one part of the large bowel are at risk of developing a further malignancy in the remainder (Bussey *et al.*, 1967; Heald and Lockhart-Mummery, 1972). The interval between the first and second (metachronous) tumour can vary between 2 and 31 years with an average interval of 13.5 years. However, the cumulative risk of developing a second cancer increases with time after first occurrence and reaches about 5 per cent after 25 years. The risk also varies depending on whether or not adenomatous (tubular) polyps or villous adenomas were present at the time of the first operation. If polyps were present at the time of the first operation – and more than one patient in five (Morson, 1974) or one patient in two (Reilly *et al.*, 1982) will have at least one associated adenoma – then the risk of recurrence reaches 10 per cent at 25 years. Although not all polyps progress to carcinomas

(Chapter 1), the increased risk of malignancy associated with them is confirmed by the number of patients who present with synchronous malignancies in neighbouring polyps and the number of individuals who intially present with benign polyps and eventually develop malignancies (Brahme *et al.*, 1974).

History of inflammatory bowel disease

Ulcerative colitis

Unlike some of the polyposis syndromes, most patients with colitis do not develop carcinoma of the large bowel. However, patients with colitis are associated with a 5–10 times increased risk of colorectal carcinoma when compared with the general population. The risk is dependent on both the extent of the disease and the length of the history. Carcinoma generally only develops in those patients where the colitis involves most of the large intestine (McDougall, 1964; de Dombal, 1966; Hulten *et al.*, 1972). Lennard-Jones *et al.* (1977), in assessing the cancer risks of 229 patients with extensive ulcerative colitis admitted to St. Mark's Hospital in London between 1966 and 1976, showed only five patients to have developed carcinoma. No carcinoma was observed in 578 patient-years of follow-up within 10 years of onset of colitis, but the risk increased to 1 in 200 patient-years in the second decade and 1 in 60 patient-years in the third decade.

Crohn's disease

Crohn's disease carries a higher than average risk of the development of carcinoma of the large bowel (Schofield, 1972; Weedon *et al.*, 1973; Gyde *et al.*, 1980; Greenstein *et al.*, 1980). In the UK and USA it is generally accepted that those individuals with long-standing (greater than 7 years' duration) Crohn's disease, regardless of age at onset, have an up to 20 times increased risk of carcinoma. Although it has been suggested that the overall risk in Crohn's disease is less than in ulcerative colitis (Gyde *et al.*, 1980), Thayer (1980) contends that it is similar.

Summary

For ease of reference the details of the conditions predisposing to colonic carcinoma are summarised in Table 2.1. Obviously, the conditions of immediate interest to the scientist are the genetically linked polyposis syndromes with an autosomal dominant mode of inheritance. For example, identification of an interstitial deletion of the long arm of chromosome 5 in FPC (FAP) patients allowed the analysis of individuals with sporadic adenocarcinomas of the colon for loss of alleles on

Table 2.1. *Summary of the conditions associated with an increased susceptibility to colorectal carcinoma*

Condition	Mode of inheritance	Distribution of polyps	Histology	Extra-intestinal manifestations	Risk of developing carcinoma
Familial polyposis coli (FPC, or FAP)	Autosomal dominant	Colon	Adenomatous polyps	None	High
Gardner's syndrome	Autosomal dominant	Colon	Adenomatous polyps	Soft tissue tumours and bone lesions	High
Peutz–Jeghers syndrome	Autosomal dominant	Entire gastro-intestinal tract except oesophagus	Hamartomatous polyps	Melanin spots on buccal mucosa, lips and digits	Low or none
Juvenile polyposis	Autosomal dominant	Usually colon and rectum but may involve small intestine and stomach	Hamartomatous polyps	None	Low or none
Turcot's syndrome	Autosomal recessive	Colon	Adenomatous polyps	Central nervous system tumours	Not certain
Colon cancer families	Autosomal recessive	Colon	Adenomatous polyps	None	Moderate
Cancer family syndrome	Autosomal dominant	Colon	Adenomatous polyps	Various adenocarcinomas, particularly of endometrium	Moderate to high
Ulcerative colitis, Crohn's disease	Possible autosomal dominant in some families	Colon	Inflammation and dysplasia	None	Low

chromosome 5. Approximately 20 per cent of tumours from patients without FPC (FAP) were shown to have allelic losses of chromosome 5 sequences (Solomon *et al.*, 1987). This suggested that becoming recessive for a gene on chromosome 5 may be a critical step in the progression of a proportion of colorectal tumours and that a locus on chromosome 5 may code for a suppressor gene in accordance with the classical theories of cancer (Knudson, 1971) and the data on retinoblastoma, another inherited cancer syndrome (Cavenee *et al.*, 1983).

The current multi-step model of colorectal tumourigenesis is one in which the steps required for the development of the tumour often involve the mutational activation of a *ras* oncogene (McCoy *et al.*, 1982; Greenhalgh and Kinsella, 1985; Bos *et al.*, 1987), coupled with the loss of several genes that normally suppress tumourigenesis (Vogelstein *et al.*, 1988; Baker *et al.*, 1989). It is important with regard to all these changes to assess their role in both 'sporadic' premalignant adenomas and in adenomas from predisposing polyposis syndromes in order to understand at which stage in the malignant progression they operate and how they might contribute to an inherited predisposition.

References

Baker, S., Fearon, E. R., Nigro, J. M., *et al.* (1989) Chromosome 17 deletions and p53 mutations in colorectal carcinomas. *Science*, **244**, 217–21.

Bartholomew, L. G., Moore, C. E., Dahlin, D. C., *et al.* (1962) Intestinal polyposis associated with mucocutaneous pigmentation. *Surg. Gynecol. Obstet.*, **115**, 1–11.

Baughman, F. A., List, C. F. and Williams, J. R. (1969) The glioma–polyposis syndrome. *New Engl. J. Med.*, **281**, 1345–6.

Bodmer, W. F., Bailey, C. J., Bodmer, J., *et al.* (1987) Localization of the gene for familial adenomatous polyposis on chromosome 5. *Nature*, **328**, 614–16.

Bonelli, L., Martines, H., Conio, M., *et al.* (1988) Family history of colorectal cancer as a risk factor for benign and malignant tumours of the large bowel: a case-control study. *Int. J. Cancer*, **41**, 513–17.

Bos, J., Fearon, E. R., Hamilton, S. R., Verlaan-de Vries, J., van Boom, J. H., van der Eb, A. J. and Vogelstein, B. (1987) Prevalence of *ras* gene mutations in human colorectal cancers. *Nature*, **327**, 293–7.

Brahme, F., Ekelund, G. R., Norden, J. R. and Wackest, A. (1974) Metachronous colorectal polyps: comparison of development of colorectal polyps and carcinomas in persons with and without histories of polyps. *Dis. Colon Rectum*, **17**, 166–71.

Burt, R. W., Bishop, D. T., Cannon, L. A., *et al.* (1985) Dominant inheritance of adenomatous colonic polyps and colorectal cancer. *New Engl. J. Med.*, **312**, 1540–4.

Bussey, H. J. R. (1975) *Familial Polyposis Coli.* Johns Hopkins University Press, Baltimore.

Bussey, H. J. R., Wallace, M. H. and Morson, B. C. (1967) Metachronous carcinoma of the large intestine and intestinal polyps. *Proc. R. Soc. Med.*, **60**, 208–10.

Camiel, M. R., Mule, J. E., Alexander, L. L. and Benninghoff, D. L. (1968) Association of thyroid carcinoma in Gardner's syndrome in siblings. *New Engl. J. Med.*, **278**, 1058–9.

Case Records of Massachussetts General Hospital (1975) Case 24. *New Engl. J. Med.*, **292**, 1340–5.

Cavenee, W. K., Dryja, T. P., Phillips, R. A., *et al.*, (1983) Expression of recessive alleles by chromosomal mechanisms in retinoblastoma. *Nature*, **305**, 779–84.

Cole, J. W. and Holden, W. D. (1959) Post-colectomy regression of adenomatous polyps of the rectum. *Arch. Surg.*, **79**, 385–92.

Cole, J. W., McKalen, A. and Powell, J. (1961) The role of ileal contents in the spontaneous regression of rectal adenomas. *Dist. Colon Rectum*, **4**, 413–18.

Crail, H. W. (1949) Multiple primary malignancies arising in rectum, brain and thyroid. *US Navy Med. Bull.*, **49**, 123–38.

deDombal, F. T., Watts, J. McK., Watkinson, G. and Coligher, J. C. (1966) Local complications of ulcerative colitis: structure, pseudo-polyposis and carcinoma of the colon and rectum. *Br. Med. J.*, **1**, 442–7.

Dozois, R. R., Judd, E. S., Dahlin, D. C., *et al.* (1969) The Peutz–Jeghers syndrome: is there a predisposition to the development of intestinal malignancy? *Arch. Surg.*, **98**, 509–17.

Dunstone, G. H. and Knaggs, T. W. L. (1972) Familial cancer of the colon and rectum. *J. Med. Genet.*, **9**, 451–6.

Erbe, R. W. (1976) Inherited gastrointestinal-polyposis syndromes. *New Engl. J. Med.*, **294**, 1101–4.

Gardner, E. J. (1951) A genetic and clinical study of intestinal polyposis, a predisposing factor for carcinoma of the colon and rectum. *Am. J. Hum. Genet.*, **3**, 167–76.

Gardner, E. J. (1962) Follow-up study of family group exhibiting dominant inheritance for syndrome including intestinal polyps, osteomas, fibromas and epidermal cysts. *Am. J. Hum. Genet.*, **14**, 376–90.

Gathright, J. B. and Cofer, T. W. (1974) Familial incidence of juvenile polyposis colis. *J. Med. Genet.*, **3**, 5–16.

Goodman, Z. D., Yardley, J. H. and Milligan, F. D. (1979) Pathogenesis of colonic polyps in multiple juvenile polyposis. *Cancer*, **43**, 1906–13.

Greenhalgh, D. A. and Kinsella, A. R. (1985) c-Ha-*ras* not c-Ki-*ras* activation in three colon tumour cell lines. *Carcinogenesis*, **6**, 1533–5.

Greenstein, A. J., Sachar, D. B., Smith, H., Janowitz, H. D. and Arfses, A. H. (1980) Patterns of neoplasia in Crohn's disease and ulcerative colitis. *Cancer*, **46**, 403–7.

Gyde, S. N., Prior, P., McCourtney, J. C., Thompson, H., Waterhouse, J. H. and Allan, R. N. (1980) Malignancy in Crohn's disease. *Gut*, **21**, 1024–9.

Haggitt, R. C. and Pitcock, J. A. (1970) Familial juvenile polyposis of the colon. *Cancer*, **26**, 1232–8.

Harned, R. K. and Williams, S. M. (1982) Familial polyposis coli and periampullary malignancy. *Dis. Colon Rectum*, **25**, 227–9.

Heald, R. J. and Lockhart-Mummery, H. E. (1972) The lesion of the second cancer of the large bowel. *Br. J. Surg.*, **59**, 16–19.

Heizelmann, F. (1964) A cancer-prone family: discussion of the question of inheritability of colonic carcinoma. *Helv. Chir. Acta*, **31**, 316–24.

Hulten, L., Kwenter, J. and Ahren, C. (1972) Precancer and carcinoma in chronic ulcerative colitis. *Scand. J. Gastroenterol.*, **7**, 663–9.

Jarvik, L. F. and Falek, A. F. (1962) Comparative data on cancer in aging twins. *Cancer*, **15**, 1009–18.

Johnson, C. D. and Thomson, H. (1986) Six synchronous colonic cancers in a pair of monozygotic twins. *Dis. Colon Rectum*, **29**, 745–6.

Kluge, T. (1964) Familial cancer of the colon. *Acta. Chir. Scand.*, **127**, 392–8.

Knudson, A. G. (1971) Mutation and cancer: statistical study of retinoblastoma. *Proc. Natl. Acad. Sc. USA*, **68**, 820–3.

Lennard-Jones, J. E., Morson, B. C., Ritchie, J. K., Shove, D. C. and Williams, C. B. (1977) Cancer in colitis: assessment of the individual risk by clinical and histological criteria. *Gastroenterology*, **73**, 1280–9.

Lovett, E. (1976) Family studies in cancer of the colon and rectum. *Por. J. Surg.*, **63**, 13–18.

Lynch, H. T. and Krush, A. J. (1967) Heredity and adenocarcinoma of the colon. *Gastroenterology*, **53**, 517–27.

Lynch, P. M. and Lynch, H. T. (eds) (1985) *Colon Cancer Genetics*. Van Nostrand Rheinhold, New York.

Lynch, H. T. and Lynch, J. (1987) Cancer predictability and minimal cancer clues in Lynch syndrome: II. *Dis. Colon Rectum*, **30**, 243–6.

Lynch, P. M., Lynch, H. T. and Harris, R. E. (1977) Hereditary proximal colonic cancer. *Dis. Colon Rectum*, **20**, 661–8.

Lynch, H. T., Lynch, P. M., Follett, K. L. and Harris, R. E. (1979) Familial polyposis coli: heterogeneous polyp expression in 2 kindreds. *J. Med. Genet.*, **16**, 1–7.

Lynch, H. T., Kimberling, W., Albano, W. A., *et al.* (1985) Hereditary non-polyposis colorectal cancer (Lynch syndrome I and II). *Cancer*, **56**, 934–8.

McCoy, M. S., Toole, J., Cunningham, J. M., Chang, E. H., Lowy, D. R. and Weinberg, R. A. (1983) Characterisation of a colon/lung carcinoma oncogene. *Nature*, **302**, 79–81.

McDougall, I. P. M. (1964) The cancer risk in ulcerative colitis. *Lancet*, **2**, 655–8.

Macklin, M. T. (1960) Inheritance of cancer of the stomach and large intestine in man. *J. Natl. Cancer Inst.*, **24**, 551–71.

Mathis, M. (1962) Familial carcinoma of the colon: a family tree from the Canton of Argau. *Schweiz. Med. Wochenschr.*, **92**, 1673–8.

Mecklin, J.-P. (1987) Frequency of hereditary colorectal carcinoma. *Gastroenterology*, **93**, 1021–5.

Mecklin, J.-P. (1989) Premalignant conditions of the gastrointestinal tract. Hereditary non-polyposis colorectal carcinoma: cancer family syndrome. *Ann. Med.*, **21**, 313–16.

Morson, B. C. (1962) Precancerous lesions of the colon and rectum: classification and controversial issues. *JAMA*, **179**, 316–21.

Morson, B. C. (1974) The polyp–cancer sequence in the large bowel. *Proc. R. Soc. Med.*, **67**, 451–7.

Morson, B. C. (1976) Genesis of colorectal cancer. *Clin. Gastroenterol.*, **3**, 505–25.

Mulvihill, J. J. (1983) The frequency of hereditary bowel cancer. In: *Prevention of Hereditary Bowel Cancer*, ed. J. P. Ingall and A. J. Mastromarino, pp. 61–75. A. R. Liss, New York.

Neel, J. V. (1954) Problems in the estimation of the frequency of uncommon inherited traits. *Am. J. Human Genet.*, **6**, 51–60.

Pierce, E. R. (1968) Some genetic aspects of familial multiple polyposis of the colon in a kindred of 1422 members. *Dis. Colon Rectum*, **11**, 321–9.

Reed, T. E. and Neel, J. V. (1955) A genetic study of multiple polyposis of the colon (with an appendix with a method of estimating relative fitness). *Am. J. Hum. Genet.*, **7**, 236–63.

Reilly, J. C., Rusin, L. C. and Theuerkauf, F. J. (1982) Colonoscopy: its role in cancer of the colon and rectum. *Dis. Colon Rectum*, **25**, 532–8.

Roth, S. I. and Helwig, E. B. (1963) Juvenile polyps of the colon and rectum. *Cancer*, **16**, 468–79.

Rozen, P. and Baratz, M. (1982) Familial juvenile colonic polyposis with associated colon cancer. *Cancer*, **49**, 1500–3.

Sachatello, C. R., Hahn, I. S. and Carrington, C. B. (1974) Juvenile gastrointestinal polyposis in a female infant: report of a case and review of the literature of a recently recognised syndrome. *Surgery*, **75**, 107–14.

Savage, D. (1956) A family history of uterine and gastrointestinal cancer. *Br. Med. J.*, **2**, 341–3.

Schofield, P. F. (1972) Intestinal malignancy and Crohn's disease. *Proc. R. Soc. Med.*, **65**, 783–4.

Smilow, P. C., Pryor, C. A. and Swinton, N. W. (1966) Juvenile polyposis coli. *Dis. Colon Rectum*, **9**, 248–54.

Smith, W. G. (1958) Gardner's syndrome and desmoid tumours. *Dis. Colon Rectum*, **1**, 323–32.

Smith, W. G. (1968) Familial multiple polyposis: research tool for investigating the aetiology of carcinoma of the colon. *Dis. Colon Rectum*, **11**, 17–31.

Solomon, E., Voss, R., Hall, V., *et al.* (1987) Chromosome 5 allele loss in human colorectal carcinomas. *Nature*, **328**, 616–19.

Stauffer, J. Q. (1973) Heritable multiple polyposis syndromes of the gastrointestinal tract. In: *Gastrointestinal Disease*, ed. M. H. Sleisenger and J. S. Fordtran, pp. 1051–60. Saunders, Philadelphia.

Stemper, T. J., Kent, T. H. and Summers, R. W. (1975) Juvenile polyposis and gastrointestinal carcinoma. *Ann. Intern. Med.*, **83**, 639–46.

Thayer, W. R. (1980)) Malignancy in inflammatory bowel disease. In: *Inflammatory Bowel Disease*, ed. J. B. Kisner and R. G. Sherker, pp. 265–78. Lea and Febiger, Philadelphia.

Turcot, J., Despres, J. P. and St Pierre, F. (1959) Malignant tumours of the central nervous system associated with familial polyposis of the colon. *Dis. Colon Rectum*, **2**, 465–8.

Veale, A. M. O. (1965) *Intestinal Polyposis*. Eugenics Laboratory Memoirs Series 40. Cambridge University Press, Cambridge.

Veale, A. M. O., McColl, I., Bussey, H. J., *et al.* (1966) Juvenile polyposis coli. *J. Med. Genet.*, **3**, 5–16.

Vogelstein, B., Fearon, E. R., Hamilton, S. R., *et al.* (1988) Genetic alterations during colorectal tumour development. *New Engl. J. Med.*, **319**, 525–32.

Warthin, A. S. (1913) Heredity with reference to carcinoma. *Arch. Intern. Med. (Chicago)*, **12**, 546–55.

Warthin, A. S. (1925) The further study of a cancer family. *J. Cancer Res.*, **9**, 279–86.

Weedon, D. D., Shorter, R. G., Illstrup, D. M., Huizenga, K. A. and Taylor, W. F. (1973) Crohn's disease and cancer. *New Engl. J. Med.*, **289**, 1099–103.

Whitehead, S. (1980) Site-specific carcinoma in identical twins. *Postgrad. Med. J.*, **56**, 69–70.

Winkler, H., Kott, I. and Reiss, R. (1983) Site-specific, simultaneous presentation of colonic carcinoma in identical twins. *Dis. Colon Rectum*, **26**, 344–6.

Woolf, C. M. (1958) A genetic study of carcinoma of the large intestine. *Am. J. Hum. Genet.*, **10**, 42–7.

Woolf, C. M., Richards, R. C. and Gardner, E. J. (1955) Occasional discrete polyps of the colon and rectum showing an inherited tendency in a kindred. *Cancer*, **8**, 403–8.

3

Epidemiology and aetiology

In the UK and the USA the incidence and mortality rates for colorectal carcinoma are second only to those of lung cancer. In the UK in 1984, there were 27 829 new cases diagnosed which accounted for 11 per cent of all newly diagnosed cancers and 13 per cent of cancer deaths (CRC Factsheet 8.2, 1988). In the USA in 1985, 138 000 new cases were diagnosed which accounted for approximately 15 per cent of all newly diagnosed cancers and 13 per cent of cancer deaths (Ziegler *et al.*, 1986). The worldwide incidence of colorectal cancer varies 20-fold or more from one part of the world to another and is highest in Australia, the USA, New Zealand and Canada (see Fig. 3.1). The incidence is greatest in developed countries (with the exception of Japan), intermediate in Eastern Europe, and lowest in Africa, Asia and South Amercia (for reviews see Burkitt, 1971; Reddy *et al.*, 1978; Reddy, 1980; Zaridze, 1983; Faivre *et al.*, 1985).

The epidemiology of colorectal cancer is interesting for two reasons: (1) because of its high incidence in so-called affluent Western societies, and (2) because the risk can be altered during a person's lifetime as evidenced by the sometimes dramatic changes in risk that accompany the changes in lifestyle which occur as a consequence of population migration. This is further exemplified by the differences in colorectal carcinoma incidence concomitant with the different lifestyles of specialised groups of individuals within the same geographic location. Although some of the international variation in colorectal carcinoma incidence may be due to genetic variation, the overwhelming body of evidence, particularly from migrant groups who have emigrated from areas of low risk to geographic areas where the population is at higher risk, indicate that colorectal carcinoma for the most part does not relate to genetic factors as much as to environmental and lifestyle factors. Moreover, it should be mentioned, when discussing geographical and regional variations, that the incidence

Fig. 3.1. Average annual incidence of colorectal carcinoma per 100 000 for men and women between the ages of 60 and 75 years worldwide (data from *Cancer Incidence in Five Continents*, vol. V, IARC, 1988).

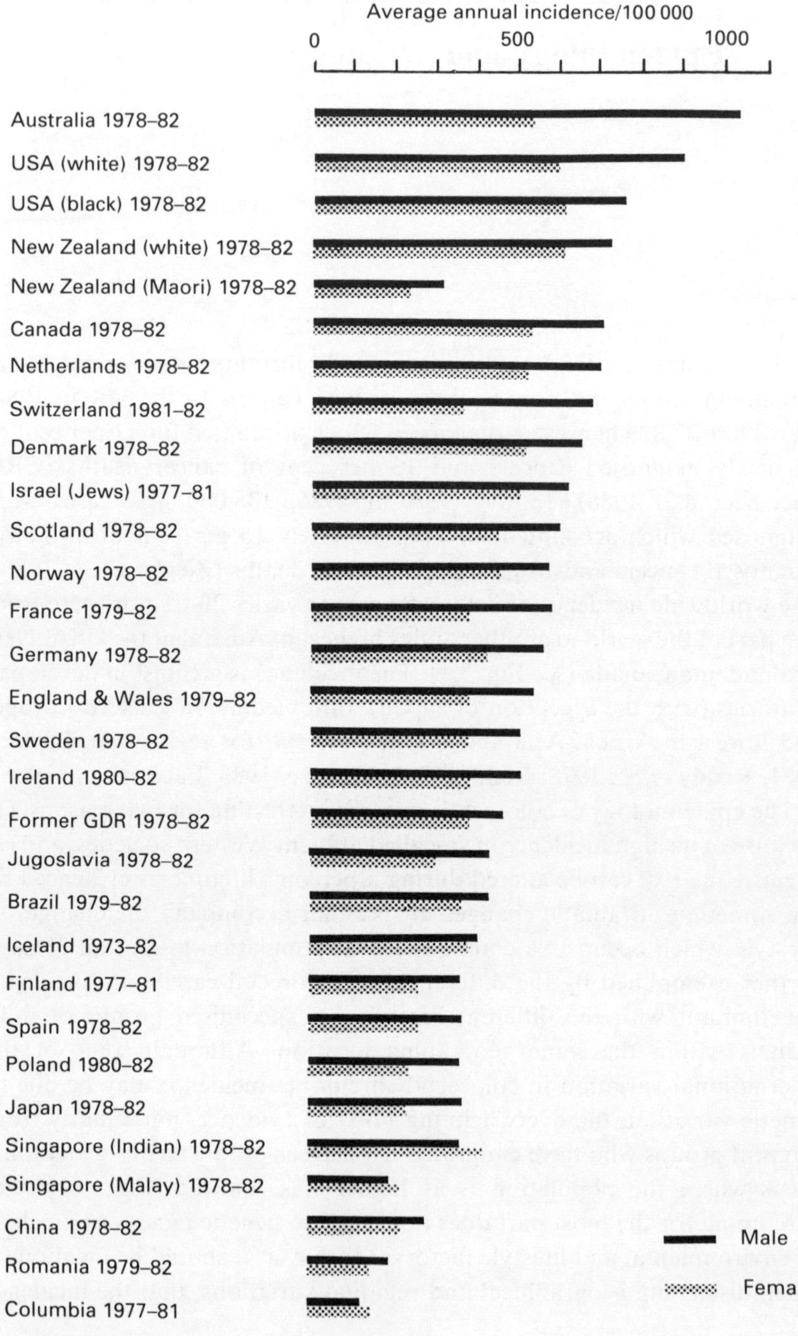

of colorectal carcinoma closely parallels the incidence of adenomatous polyps in the population as discussed in the previous chapter (Correa and Haenszel, 1978).

Population studies

Geographic distribution

A network of cancer registries throughout the world has led to a series of publications by the International Agency for Research on Cancer (IARC) entitled *Cancer Incidence in Five Continents*. The highest incidence is reported in New Zealand, the USA, Canada and Scotland, whilst the rates are generally low in Africa, Asia and South America. Europe assumes an intermediate position although Western Europe and Scandinavia generally have higher incidences than Eastern Europe. Of the developed countries Japan and Finland provide exceptions, being highly industrialised but with a low incidence of large bowel cancer (see Fig. 3.1). There are also substantial regional variations which will be discussed in detail later. For example the incidence of colorectal carcinoma in Denmark is three times that in certain regions of Finland, and in Britain, Sweden, the USA and India there are regional variations within the individual countries. Also, it should be mentioned here that there is a strong correlation between the incidence rates for the two classical subdivisions of the large bowel: the colon and rectum. With very few exceptions the colon–rectum ratios are close to unity. Lower ratios are seen in Romania and Jugoslavia due to a deficit of colon carcinoma, and the opposite extreme is represented by Jamaica where the incidence of colon carcinoma is twice that of the rectum. Switzerland and countries with a very high incidence of large bowel carcinoma overall have high rates of colon carcinoma. Thus, for the purposes of this chapter and the book as a whole, colon carcinoma and rectal carcinoma will be classified together as colorectal carcinoma, unless specifically separated.

Migrant studies

In general, as groups of people move to new geographic locations their risk for various cancers shifts from that of their country of origin towards that of their host country (Haenszel, 1982). A mortality study of Japanese-Americans (both native and foreign born) during the period 1949–1952 showed that the rates of colorectal carcinoma among US Japanese were lower than amongst US whites and higher than amongst the Japanese in Japan (Smith, 1956). Furthermore, the increased rate was more prevalent amongst the male US Japanese population. A decade later (1959–1962) the colorectal mortality rates for the US Japanese had moved

Table 3.1. *Standardised mortality ratios (SMRs) for cancer of the colon and rectum in US Japanese (Haenszel and Kurihara, 1968)*

		Colon		Rectum	
SMRs for US Japanese	Year	Male	Female	Male	Female
Relative to whites	1949–52	0.67	0.34	0.80	0.65
	1959–62	0.70	0.46	0.95	0.63
Relative to Japanese	1949–52	3.71	1.74	1.37	0.91
	1959–62	3.46	2.11	1.34	0.69

even closer to the US white rates (Haenszel and Kurihara, 1968; Table 3.1) and by 1968–1972 the colon cancer incidence rates for Japanese men and women in Hawaii up to 70 years of age were similar to those for the white population, but were lower for those Japanese over 70 years of age. This difference for the Hawaiian populations can be explained on the basis that most Japanese Hawaiians aged less than 70 at the time of the study were the children of migrants, whilst those aged over 70 represented the migrant population (Correa and Haenszel, 1978).

Colorectal carcinoma risks have also been studied amongst the Chinese-American population, although this has been complicated by the striking risk variations within China. The 1970 age-adjusted mortality rates for colorectal carcinoma amongst foreign-born Chinese-American men and women were 5.6 and 2.7 times the respective rates in Guangzhou province from where they emigrated. The incidence rates for the Hong Kong Chinese living in Hong Kong are already 3 times those for Guangzhou province (Ziegler *et al.*, 1986). Analysis of the Puerto Ricans living in New York showed the rates to be almost twice those in Puerto Rico, but only half to two-thirds those of New York whites (Monk and Warshauer, 1975). European migrants to the US assumed the US rates within one generation (Haenszel, 1961), whilst Mexicans reached only 50 per cent of the US rate in the first generation. In all instances the migrant colorectal mortality rates did not reach those of the USA as frequently for women as for men and presumably reflected differences in the degree of acculturation. Similar patterns of increased risk were observed for the Polish, Jugoslavian, Greek, Italian and Chinese populations that migrated to Australia (McMichael *et al.*, 1980). Only the Polish population reached the risk rates of the native Australian population, whilst Chinese males acquired a higher risk than the native Australian white population of New South Wales (Zhang *et al.*, 1984). Conversely, Scottish and English migrants to Australia have shown a decreased risk consistent with

Table 3.2. *Age-adjusted incidence per 100 000 of colon and rectal cancer in Israel 1973–1977 (Ziegler* et al., *1986)*

Population	Males Colon	Males Rectum	Females Colon	Females Rectum
Jews born in Europe or USA	14.5	13.9	14.4	13.4
Jews born in Africa or Asia	6.8	5.7	5.5	4.6
Jews born in Israel	13.6	11.7	10.0	9.5
Non-Jews	3.3	3.1	1.8	1.5

migration from an area of higher risk to an area of lower risk. A decreased risk is also seen in Israel, where on the basis of the 1973–1977 age-adjusted incidence rates (Waterhouse *et al.*, 1982), Israeli-born Jews had a risk of colorectal carcinoma below that of European- or American-born Israelis but above that of Israelis born in Africa or Asia (Table 3.2). Similar trends are seen in England and Wales, where colon cancer amongst males is seen to increase in immigrants from lower-risk areas such as Pakistan, Sri Lanka and Poland and to decrease in American immigrants from high-risk areas (see Fig. 3.2; Fraser and Adelstein, 1982).

All these data suggest the importance of lifestyle factors. Further support for this idea comes from racial differences in the incidence of colorectal carcinoma between racial groups occupying the same geographical area. For example, the colon cancer incidence in Hawaii

Fig. 3.2. Mortality from colon carcinoma amongst the male immigrant population in England and Wales 1970–1972 (after Fraser and Adelstein, 1982).

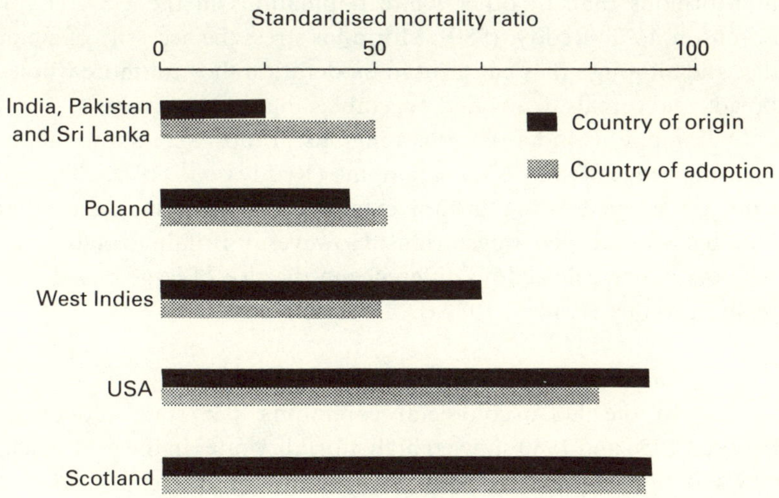

amongst Hawaiians and Filipinos is low compared with that for Caucasians, Japanese or Chinese. Further evidence of racial differences in colorectal carcinoma come from New Zealand where there is a 2- to 3-fold difference between non-Maoris and Maoris, and from Singapore where the incidence is 3 times higher in the Chinese than in the Malayan or Indian populations (Waterhouse *et al.*, 1982). Racial differences are presumably markers or determinants of cultural and therefore lifestyle differences.

Religion and lifestyle

Newill (1961) investigated cancer mortality among whites of different religions in New York City. Jewish men and women had respectively 1.37 and 1.24 times the risk of colon cancer of New York Catholics and Protestants, whose risks were the same. The risk of rectal cancer was apparently not influenced by religion in the same way. Subsequent studies of Russian-born immigrants in New York City, upstate New York and the USA in general showed a large percentage of these populations to be Jewish and, consistent with this, to exhibit an elevated risk of colon carcinoma (Seidman, 1970, 1971; Haenszel, 1971; Greenwald *et al.*, 1975).

Also in the USA, the mortality from colorectal carcinoma amongst Seventh Day Adventists living in California is substantially lower (60 per cent) than amongst the general population (Phillips *et al.*, 1980). It is claimed that the Seventh Day Adventists consume virtually no meat and follow a lacto-ovo-vegetarian diet containing no poultry or fish but including milk products and eggs. Similarly colorectal carcinoma is lower in Mormons than in other white populations in the USA (Lyon and Sorenson, 1978; Reddy, 1980). Mormons stress the necessity of a balanced diet and although they eat meat in moderation they eat more whole-grain breads and cereals, fruits and vegetables than other groups.

In Bombay in India, various religious groups were shown to vary in their incidence of colorectal carcinoma (Reddy *et al.*, 1978). The Parsees, who are a meat-eating group, exhibited a higher incidence than the Hindus, who are lacto-vegetarians. However in Britain a study of nuns in religious orders showed no difference in the risk of large bowel cancer in relation to diet (Kinlen, 1982a).

Socioeconomic influences

In the USA colorectal carcinoma per state economic area between 1950 and 1980 showed high mortality rates in the north-east, with elevated rates in upstate New York and western Pennsylvania, Ohio,

Indiana and Illinois. In general rates in the southern USA, where there were a higher percentage of blacks in the population, remained significantly lower than for the general US population. The elevated risk in the north-eastern and northern-central states of the USA was thought to be due to increased urbanisation and the higher socioeconomic status of these groups (Haenszel and Dawson, 1965; Ziegler *et al.*, 1986). Blot and colleagues (1976) observed positive correlations for both sexes with county, income and median years of education.

Colorectal carcinoma is generally considered to be a disease of affluent economically developed countries. In almost every country where regional studies have been carried out on genetically homogeneous populations, wide differences have been found in the local levels of incidence (as assessed by either mortality or registration data) which can be explained on socioeconomic grounds. In Cali in Columbia, the risk of carcinoma was 4 times greater in the upper than the lower socioeconomic classes for both sexes and for all age groups (Armstrong and Doll, 1975). A higher prevalence amongst the higher socioeconomic groups has also been noted for Hong Kong (Committee on Diet, Nutrition and Cancer, 1982) and Japan (Wynder and Reddy, 1978). This is not true in the UK where higher mortality is seen amongst the lower socioeconomic groups.

In England recent evidence from cancer statistics (registrations) in England and Wales and the Office of Population Censuses and Surveys (OPCS) shows that the incidence of colorectal cancer in both sexes is above average in the North West Region, Northern England in general, and the West Midlands. Rectal carcinoma is particularly high in Wales. In all instances, however, mortality from colorectal carcinoma is higher in the conurbations and more densely populated areas than in the smaller towns and more rural areas. Male mortality from rectal carcinoma exhibits a clear social class gradient with higher mortality in the lower social classes, whilst for colon carcinoma there is very little difference. For married women whose social status is determined by their husbands occupation, the mortality from rectal carcinoma is the same as for men. However, in the case of colon carcinoma the mortality is higher in the three lower social classes and in social class 1 (Fraser and Adelstein, 1982).

Conclusions

Epidemiological studies relating to colorectal carcinoma reveal geographic, ethnic and regional differences in the distribution of the disease. They show changes in mortality over time and after migration, a higher risk in urban populations and generally a higher mortality amongst males. The more specific conclusions are as follows:

1. The risk of colorectal carcinoma shows a wide geographic variation.
2. The risk can increase or decrease within a migrating population within a single generation and the change in risk is much more rapid than for other major cancers within a migrating population.
3. The risk of colorectal carcinoma can vary between certain specialised populations on specialised diets.
4. The risk is clearly related to race (culture), reinforcing the importance of lifestyle factors.
5. Even within the same cultural framework, for example the white population of Britain, there are large regional variations.

Since, as discussed in Chapter 2, genetic factors account for a very small proportion of colorectal carcinomas, these observations suggest that the most important lifestyle factor with respect to colorectal carcinoma risk is diet. Furthermore, the studies of migrant populations even suggest that the risk is principally determined by adult diet (e.g the Florida migration studies: Ziegler *et al.*, 1986) and more by recent events than remote experiences.

Dietary studies

Epidemiologists, having surmised that diet is the lifestyle factor responsible for the large variations in the risk of acquiring colorectal carcinoma, still have not identified the critical components responsible for reducing or increasing the risk. The risk is thought to be increased in populations on high-fat, high-meat diets (Fig. 3.3), with consumption of beer, spirits, wine and cigarettes also contributing to an increase in risk. On the other hand, the risk appears to be decreased in populations with diets high in vegetables and fibre. Other contributing factors are thought to be differences in the bacterial gut flora and the presence of trace elements. Colorectal carcinoma is remarkable in that it is one of the commonest tumours for which there is no specific occupational factor.

Dietary fat

Studies of the Seventh Day Adventists in California (Phillips *et al.*, 1980) and the Parsees and Hindus in Bombay (Reddy *et al.*, 1978) suggested that low-fat vegetarian diets were protective. Most of the fat in the Western diet comes from meat and, in fact, the data showing the correlation between colon carcinoma incidence in women and per capita daily meat consumption (Fig 3.3a) correlate better with the data for worldwide incidence of colon carcinoma than do the data for total dietary fat (Fig 3.3b). Wynder and Shigematsu as long ago as 1967 suggested that colon cancer was associated with dietary fat. Drasar and Irving (1973) compared dietary data and the incidence of colon cancer from 37 countries and showed the incidence of colorectal cancer to be strongly

Fig. 3.3. (*a*) Colon cancer incidence per 100 000 women in different countries worldwide as a function of their per capita meat consumption (Armstrong and Doll, 1975). (*b*) Colon cancer mortality per 100 000 of the population in different countries worldwide as a function of daily fat consumption (after Wynder, 1987).

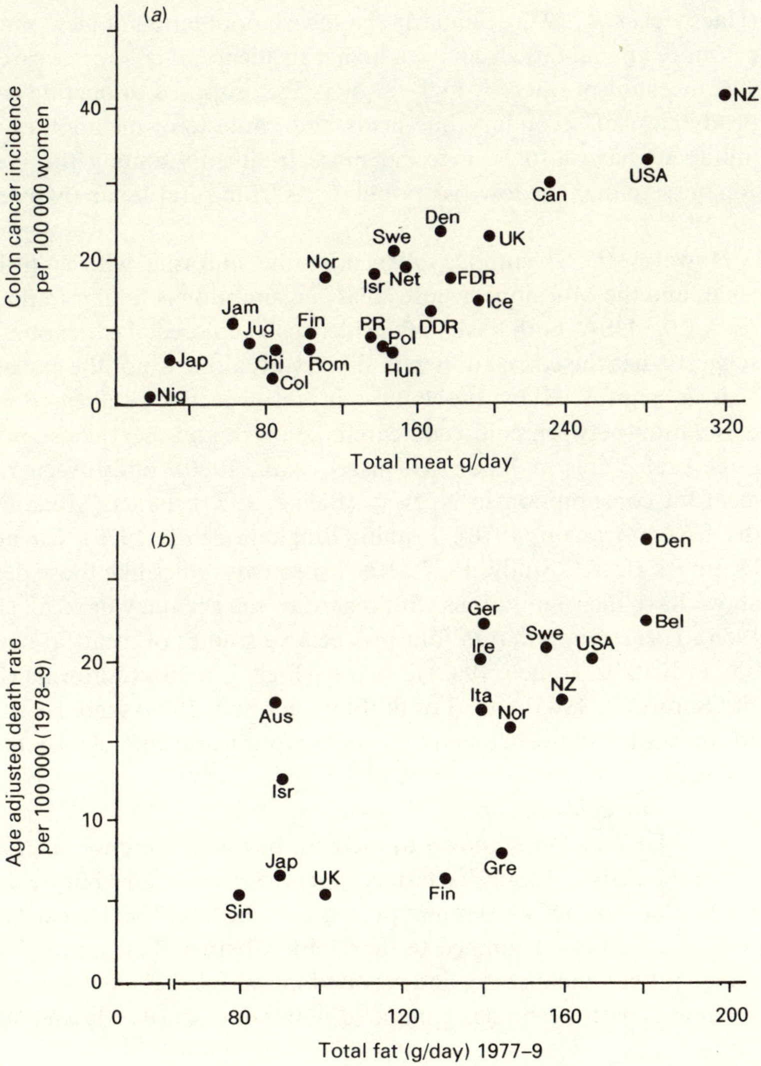

correlated with the intake of combined fat and animal protein, but not vegetable fat.

Greece, Japan and Finland occupy unique positions for developed countries (Fig. 3.3). In Japan this could be attributed to the low saturated fat consumption and in Greece to the fact that olive oil, a monosaturated fat, is the principal fat used (Wynder, 1987). In Finland, however, where the diet is high in dairy fats, other dietary components are considered to contribute a protective effect. Furthermore, as discussed earlier, Japanese immigrants to Hawaii who are known to have a much higher fat intake than the Japanese in Japan have an increased risk of colorectal carcinoma (Haenszel *et al.*, 1973). Similarly the Jewish population of New York, who eat more animal fat, also have a higher incidence of colorectal carcinoma. The mechanism whereby high-fat diets are proposed to operate is via the production of secondary bile acids and cholesterol metabolites. Faecal mutagens have also been found more frequently among the Hawaiian Japanese than in the low-risk populations from rural Japan (Mower *et al.*, 1982).

However, the Seventh Day Adventists of California, who eat little or no meat, and the Mormons, whose meat consumption is similar to that of the rest of the USA, both have low incidences of colorectal carcinoma, which suggests that the correlation with dietary fat alone is not the explanation. This is reinforced by the failure in retrospective studies to show a correlation between colorectal carcinoma risk and meat consumption in three prefectures in Japan (Haenszel *et al.*, 1980), or between risk and meat/fat consumption in Norway (Bjelke, 1973), Israel (Modan, 1975), the USA (Graham, 1978), Britain (Bingham *et al.*, 1979), Finland and Denmark (IARC Study, 1977). Retrospective studies like those described above have their limitations with regard to the accuracy of recall (Kinlen, 1986). It is striking that in four prospective studies of meat/fat consumption in Britain (Kinlen, 1982), Norway (Bjelke, 1973), California (Phillips and Snowdon, 1983) and Hawaii (Stemmerman, 1984) there is absolutely no correlation between dietary fat consumption and colorectal carcinoma.

Bile acids

Dietary fat is known to increase bile acid secretion, increase the metabolic activity of gut bacteria and increase secondary bile acids in the colon that can act as tumour promoters (Hill, 1975). Faecal bile acid profiles have been examined to determine whether they are predictive of malignant colonic disease, and elevated faecal bile acid levels were found in patients with adenomas compared with controls (Reddy and Wynder,

1977). Patients with colon carcinoma were reported to excrete more total faecal bile than other groups and a correlation between bile acid excretion and adenoma size has been postulated (Hill *et al.*, 1978, 1983). However, the faecal bile profiles for individuals with or without adenomas or carcinomas are identical and it seems more likely, extrapolating from *in vitro* studies, that bile acids are responsible for promoting the expression of colonic epithelium that is already neoplastically altered.

Cholesterol

The suspicion that high cholesterol intake might be a risk factor for colorectal carcinoma came from the observation that a strong correlation existed between the international mortality rates for colorectal carcinoma and those for heart disease (Wynder and Shigematsu, 1967). Raised levels of faecal cholesterol have been associated with increased risk in international and regional comparisons of low- and high-risk groups (Hill *et al.*, 1971, Reddy and Wynder, 1973, Liu *et al.*, 1979). Healthy, low-risk Americans consuming a mixed Western diet excreted higher levels than low-risk South African blacks (Salyers *et al.*, 1977); also those individuals with predisposing diseases, namely FAP (Reddy *et al.*, 1976), adenomatous polyps (Reddy and Wynder, 1977), ulcerative colitis (Reddy and Wynder, 1977) and Gardner's syndrome (Core and Watne, 1974), all excreted more cholesterol and metabolites than their corresponding control groups.

Surprisingly, however, colorectal patients have low serum cholesterol levels (Rose and Shipley, 1980; Kark *et al.*, 1980) and two studies showed serum cholesterol to be low in individuals for many years before diagnosis of cancer when compared with non-cancer controls (Sorlie and Feinlieb, 1982; Schatzkin *et al.*, 1987). However, the cholesterol controversy continues, because the results of major trials involving diet and cholesterol-lowering drugs (McMichael *et al.*, 1984) suggest that there is little difference between cancer incidence and mortality in treated and non-treated groups. In contrast, two recent publications both report a positive correlation between serum cholesterol and colorectal carcinoma in men (Tornberg *et al.*, 1986) and adenoma formation in women (Mannes *et al.*, 1986). Finally, a study of serum cholesterol levels, coronary heart disease and cancer in Scotland (Isles *et al.*, 1989) showed a positive correlation of cholesterol level with heart disease and a negative correlation with cancer in men. However, although the negative correlation between cholesterol and cancer in general was very strong, the effect for colorectal cancer was hardly significant.

Dietary fibre

For a long time a negative relationship has been indicated between colorectal carcinoma risk and dietary fibre (DF). Burkitt (1971) attributed the high incidence of colon cancer in Western societies to a lack of fibre in the diet. Western diets include large amounts of animal protein, meat, fat, sugar and highly refined cereal products and low amounts of fibre. As a result transit time through the large intestine is slowed, alllowing more time for gut bacteria to degrade intraluminal components, produce carcinogens or co-carcinogens and enable such carcinogens to interact with the intestinal mucosa (Burkitt *et al.*, 1972).

Dietary fibre is the part of the ingested plant material resistant to digestive enzymes, resulting in an increase in faecal bulk. There is evidence to suggest that the protective effect against colon cancer may be due to the absorption, dilution or metabolism of the carcinogens or co-carcinogens characteristic of the Western diet by components of fibre (Reddy *et al.*, 1978). There is also evidence that certain types of fibre may bind bile acids, affect the metabolism of bile salts and increase the faecal excretion of these compounds. Thus, dietary fibre may prevent or reduce the toxic effects of certain metabolites or carcinogens (Freeman, 1979; Sian, 1987). Fibre is also believed to reduce the formation of potential tumour promoters and dilute any such co-carcinogens formed by its bulking effect (Reddy *et al.*, 1978). The intestinal microflora are also sensitive to changes in dietary substrate, including fibre, and may have an important role to play in colon carcinogenesis (Hill, 1974; Jain *et al.*, 1980).

Evidence for the protective effect of dietary fibre comes from the IARC co-ordinated study in Copenhagen, Denmark, and Kuopio, Finland, which compared the dietary fibre intake of the low-risk population of Kuopio with the high-risk population of Copenhagen (IARC Study, 1977). A more recent IARC co-ordinated Danish–Finnish study shows more specifically an inverse relationship between large bowel cancer and cereals and total dietary fibre (Jensen *et al.*, 1982). In Britain, Bingham *et al.* (1979) showed that a specific fraction of the dietary fibre and vegetables (other than potatoes) were protective against colon carcinoma, but later retracted the specific effect showing only an effect of fibre in general. In a metabolic epidemiology study of colon cancer, a high-risk group from New York was compared with two low-risk groups, one the rural Finns from Kuopio and the other the Japanese. The higher consumption of whole-grain cereals and breads by the Finns resulted in a higher stool bulk and lower bile acid concentrations than in the New York population, despite the fact that the levels of fat consumption in the two populations were similar (Wynder, 1987). In fact because of the higher stool bulk the concentration of bile acids in the faeces of the Finns was similar to that of the Japanese. Thus, cereal fibre was clearly protective, as bile acids have been found to act as promoters in colon carcinogenesis in rats (Reddy *et al.*, 1978). The Japanese excrete less bile acid per day and have a lower concentration in the faeces because of a lower fat intake.

A negative relationship has also been observed between colorectal carcinoma and vegetable consumption, and most studies have shown that vegetables are eaten less frequently by colon cancer patients. Malhotra (1967) noticed a difference in the colon cancer incidence between the northern and southern populations of India. Vegetable fibre was abundant in the stools of the Punjabis from the north of the country, but was completely absent in the stools of the inhabitants from the south of the country where the risk of colorectal cancer was much higher. Vegetable consumption was also seen to have a protective effect in populations from New York (Graham, 1978), Israel (Modan *et al.*, 1975), Norway (Bjelke, 1980), Britain (Bingham *et al.*, 1979), Greece (Manousos *et al.*, 1983) and Singapore (Lee *et al.*, 1989). In Britain, 40 per cent of the fibre consumed in the diet comes from vegetables and one candidate for the protective effect provided by vegetables is beta-carotene. Certainly the ingestion of cabbage, carotene-rich vegetables, and cruciferous vegetables such as cauliflower, broccoli and Brussels sprouts, has been shown to have an inverse relationship with colorectal carcinoma. In fact vitamin A has been shown to provide a protective effect against a variety of cancers (Peto *et al.*, 1981).

As for dietary fat, the risk of colorectal carcinoma could be correlated with vegetable consumption for some countries but not others (Haenszel *et al.*, 1973). Also, a poor correlation was reported between average intake of crude fibre and colon cancer risk in different countries (Armstrong and Doll, 1975). However, these discrepancies are probably quite simply due to differences in the definitions used for fibre in the diet. Until recently (Slattery *et al.* 1988), no population-based colon cancer studies have examined the defined chemical components of fibre. Insoluble dietary fibres (IDF) such as cellulose, lignin and some hemicellulose reduce transit time, provide bulk and dilute the faecal contents. These properties are attributable to the insoluble fibre matrix, which remains intact in the gut. On the other hand soluble dietary fibres (SDF) such as gums, pectins and other hemicelluloses have a high water-holding capacity which increases their viscosity. In addition they form gels which trap nutrients, digestive enzymes and possibly harmful bile acids. The studies with crude fibre involved the removal of all the SDF and varying amounts of IDF, leaving 50–90 per cent lignin, 10–15 per cent cellulose and 20 per cent hemicellulose (Lanza and Butrum, 1986). Studies with neutral detergent fibre involved the removal of the insoluble lignin and cellulose and most of the hemicellulose. The non-starch polysaccharides contain most of the fibre in the diet and can be further divided into cellulose polysaccharides or non-cellulose polysaccharides (Englyst and Cummings, 1986). The most common components of non-cellulose polysaccharides include pentoses and hexoses.

The study group for investigation of the effects of defined components of fibre on the risk/incidence of colorectal carcinoma was a predominantly Mormon population of Utah, most of whom were more than 60 years of age and 40–50 per cent of whom had a better than high school level of education (Slattery *et al.*, 1988). The data for Utah males showed a strong protective effect for crude fibre and an inconsistent protective effect for neutral detergent fibre and DF. In the same study for every tumour site for males, fruit consumption was shown to have a protective effect. Vegetable consumption was also protective although the magnitude of the effect was less than for fruit consumption. Contrary to the observations made in the Finnish study, grain consumption in this study did not appear to reduce the colorectal carcinoma risk. In Utah females, consumption of vegetables protected against cancers of the colon, particularly the ascending colon. The same was true for fruit consumption. No consistent observation was made between grain consumption and colon cancer. Finally, to help with the interpretation of these results Slattery *et al.* (1988) compared the various indices of fibre with the major food sources of fibre and found the highest correlation to be between crude dietary fibre and fruit and vegetables.

Bacterial flora

In 1971, Hill *et al.* reported a correlation between the mortality rates for colorectal carcinoma in certain countries and the bacteriological and chemical composition of the faeces of the different populations. Samples from countries that had a higher incidence of the disease, had a higher frequency of bacteria that could degrade bile salts. Also, stools from high-incidence countries had higher concentrations of neutral and acid sterols derived from the breakdown of cholesterol and bile salts, respectively. In fact, populations with high-fat diets appeared to have intestinal flora with a greater capacity for breaking down the more plentiful degradation products of bile salts into putative mutagens. However, there is very little doubt, except for one report (Watabe and Bernstein, 1985), that bile acids are not mutagens (Venitt *et al.*, 1987; reviewed Venitt, 1988).

More recently it has been proposed that high-fat, high-protein, low-fibre diets can cause an unfavourable microbial environment in the colon, increasing the risk of the large bowel carcinoma (McBurney *et al.*, 1987). The human colon contains more than 100 species of bacteria (Moore and Holdeman, 1974), estimated to number 10^{10}–10^{11} bacteria per gram of faecal material (Moore *et al.*, 1978). The majority of these bacterial species are anaerobic and utilise dietary fibre as an energy source. They have been shown to have inducible rather than constitutive enzyme activities (Salyers *et al.*, 1977) which can respond to changes in the composition of the colonic contents. McBurney *et al.* (1987) proposed that the typical Western diet results in the irregular propulsion of rapidly fermentable digesta into the colon. As the small amount of available carbohydrate entering the colon is rapidly depleted, a proteolytic fermentation ensues and carcinogens are concentrated into a small colonic mass and there may even be enhanced microbial degradation of colonic mucosa. This is because the rapidly proliferating microbial population soon depletes its dietary substrate and for the most part enters a stationary phase of growth. However, some microbial species seek alternative substrates and may induce the enzymes necessary to ferment glycoproteins and may ultimately therefore cause pre-cancerous lesions in the colonic epithelium. The longer this ("feast or famine") situation prevails, the more likely it is that the colonic microbial populations and fermentation end-products will promote the progression of malignant disease.

Faecal mutagens

Genotoxic agents are known to exist in human faeces (Bruce *et al.*, 1977; Kuhnlein and Kuhnlein, 1980; Kuhnlein *et al.*, 1981; Venitt, 1981, 1982*a, b*, 1988; Wilkins and Van Tassell, 1983; Reddy, 1986). In an attempt to determine the role of faecal genotoxicity in the development of large bowel cancer, the levels of faecal mutagens have been determined in donors from populations with different risk levels by employing the *Salmonella* test (Ames *et al.*, 1975; Maron and Ames, 1983). Ehrich *et al.* (1979) demonstrated that a higher percentage of high-risk white residents of Johannesburg, South Africa, produced mutagenic faeces than did age- and sex-matched low-risk urban or rural blacks. Reddy *et al.* (1980*a*) compared the faecal mutagenicity of three populations with different risks of large bowel cancer with the following results. The percentage of mutagenic faeces was 13 per cent in a low-risk population from rural Finland, none in ovo-lacto-vegetarian Seventh Day Adventists from New York and 22 per cent in a high risk omnivorous population from New York. Reddy *et al.* (1980*b*) also reported that the faeces of the high-risk

New York population were also the most co-mutagenic. Similar studies have been conducted in New Zealand and amongst the Japanese populations of Hawaii and Japan (Ferguson and Alley, 1982; Mower *et al.*, 1982), with less obvious results. In an investigation of rural and urban Finns by Reddy *et al.* (1985) there was no significant difference between the two groups for the excretion of faecal mutagens although their risks for colorectal cancer were markedly different. Detailed analysis of the diets of the donors showed that there was no significant difference in the intake of total protein, fat or calories, although the rural group consumed significantly more dietary fibre than the urban group. Reddy *et al.* (1985) claimed that irrespective of which group they came from, men who consumed more that 28 g of dietary fibre per day and women who consumed more than 24 g of dietary fibre per day produced faeces that were not mutagenic. In three studies of faecal mutagens in colon cancer patients versus matched asymptomatic controls (Bruce and Dion, 1980; Ferguson and Alley, 1982; Askew *et al.* 1982) no significant difference was observed between the two groups. Unfortunately all these studies and the studies reviewed by Venitt (1988) using the fluctuation test (Green and Muriel, 1976; Green *et al.* 1976) are subject to the limitations of the assay systems.

However, in two studies in which the subjects were given controlled diets (Hayatsu *et al.*, 1985; Venitt *et al.*, 1986) a correlation could be made between diet and faecal mutagenicity. In the first study (Hayatsu *et al.*, 1985) three healthy subjects abstained from cooked meat or fish from day 1. A meal of fried beef was taken on day 4 and consecutive stool samples collected from days 3 to 8. No further cooked meat was taken until after day 8. Faecal mutagenicity rose from almost zero on days 3 and 4, to high levels at days 5 and 6, but had fallen back to the original levels by day 8. The authors proposed that the increased faecal mutagenicity was due to metabolites of the mutagens that were identified in the fried beef. In the second study (Venitt *et al.* 1986) a healthy Caucasian male on a Western diet was monitored for faecal mutagenicity following normal, high-fat and high-fibre diets. Five out of five normal diet samples and four out of four high-fat samples were positive for mutagenicity. Only one out of four high-fibre samples was positive, demonstrating a significant difference between high-fibre and other diets.

So where do the faecal mutagens that are present come from? In the study of Hayatsu *et al.* (1985) the faecal mutagenicity resulting from the ingestion of the fried beef was only transient. The factors that govern the generation of mutagenic activity during the cooking of meat and fish have been studied in several laboratories and it has been concluded that mutagen production increases with time and temperature of cooking (Overik *et al.*, 1984; Knize *et al.*, 1985; Nagao *et al.*, 1985; Nilsson *et al.*, 1986). The pyrolysis products of proteins and amino acids are particularly well studied and several heterocyclic amines have been isolated from grilled or fried meat or fish (Nagao *et al.*, 1985; Sugimura, 1985). The relevance to colorectal cancer of faecal mutagens derived from cooked meat is difficult to judge from only one well-conducted study of three subjects (Hayatsu *et al.*, 1985). The protein and amino acid pyrolysates of the type found in fried beef are indirect mutagens that require activation. Rat colonic mucosa possesses enzyme systems capable of metabolising indirect mutagens and carcinogens to their active derivatives (Strobel and Fang, 1981). Therefore, it is reasonable to suppose that the normal human colonic mucosa is capable of metabolising a variety of substrates to their active derivatives.

Potent mutagens, called faecapentaenes, that are actually formed in the human colon have also been identified (Wilkins *et al.*, 1980; Bruce *et al.*, 1982; Hirai *et al.*, 1982). Their production is stimulated by bile and bile acids (Van Tassell *et al.*, 1982*a*) and it was suggested that bile acids resulted in the selection for increased growth of bile-resistant mutagen-producing bacteria. The five mutagen-producing species of bacteria (Van Tassell *et al.*, 1982*b*) are amongst the most common in the intestinal microflora and are present in mutagen excretors and non-excretors alike. Studies using synthetic faecapentaenes show them to be potent bacterial mutagens and to be potent inducers of point mutations in human cells in culture (Goggelman *et al.*, 1986; Plummer *et al.*, 1986). However, to date the production of faecapentaenes is dependent on the presence of a precursor whose origin and structure are unknown. The other conditions that are a prerequisite for their production are the presence of a sufficiently high concentration of bile acids, a pH above 6.0 and the presence of lysed cells from certain species of *Bacteroides* (Hirai *et al.*, 1985). The latter conditions are those that would be expected in the colon of an individual on a high-fat, low-fibre diet, which brings us back to the role of diet in the aetiology of colorectal carcinoma.

pH

Examination of the relationship between colonic cell proliferation, large bowel fermentation and experimental colon carcinogenesis showed the fermentation of dietary fibre to be associated with a reduction in the pH of the luminal contents. This increase in acidity was shown in experimental systems to be associated with an increase in the frequency and yield of tumours. However, although in dietary studies in animals fermentable fibres such as pectin and guar appeared to stimulate cell proliferation, no consistent relationship between cell proliferation and colon cancer frequency could be shown. Chronic dietary acidification of the luminal contents (Jacobs, 1986*a,b*), though, was associated with an increase in tumours of the distal colon. Overall, however, none of these experimental dietary studies strongly supports the role of an acid luminal pH in colon carcinogenesis.

In contrast, human epidemiological studies have shown an association between reduced colon cancer risk and low faecal pH (Cummings, 1985; Samelson *et al.*, 1985; Walker *et al.*, 1986), although two small case-control studies (Pietroiusti *et al.*, 1983; McDonald *et al.*, 1978) showed the faecal pH of individuals with colon cancer to be lower than that of the control group. Consistent with these latter observations, in human dietary intervention studies to study variations in faecal mutagenesis between different individuals on identical diets (reviewed by Venitt, 1988), low faecal pH appeared to correlate positively with high mutagenicity. It is obvious, therefore, that differences in luminal faecal pH reflect differences in both the diet and the bacterial flora of the large intestine and that the inter-relationships of the many factors involved is complex. The question still remains whether these factors are causative or merely indicative of an increased colorectal cancer risk.

Beer consumption

Beer drinking has been shown to be associated with colorectal carcinoma, particularly rectal carcinoma, in a variety of studies. In Liverpool, England, a significant relationship was demonstrated between the incidence of intestinal cancer and beer drinking (Stocks, 1958), whilst Bjelke (cited in Enstrom, 1977) found in a study of 12 000 men, that heavy beer-drinkers developed colorectal carcinoma more often than those who drank less beer. Enstrom (1977) correlated rectal cancer mortality with the per capital consumption of beer in different American states and demonstrated that the male to female ratio of rectal cancer mortality correlated strongly with beer consumption. Two more recent studies of mortality from rectal carcinoma amongst brewery workers who were allowed a free quota of beer, showed a significant excess of deaths from rectal cancer amongst Dublin workers (Dean *et al.*, 1979) but not amongst workers in Copenhagen (Jensen, 1979). Part of the explanation for this discrepancy could be the chemical and other differences between the stout brewed in Ireland and the lager brewed in Denmark. However, both the national consumption of beer and the national incidence of rectal carcinoma are higher in Denmark, making a distinction between the normal population and brewery workers more difficult.

Dietary minerals

Although macronutrients are heavily implicated in the aetiology of colorectal carcinoma, it is possible that micronutrients might be mediators of cancer risk (Nelson *et al.*, 1987). Selenium in the diet is found primarily in cereal grains and seafood with only low levels occurring in red meat. Epidemiological studies have demonstrated a higher cancer mortality in low selenium areas and a protective effect of selenium on cancer mortality from cancers of the colon and rectum (Schrauzer, 1978; Clark, 1985). Calcium intake is also reported to be protective. In Sweden, colon tumour incidence is inversely proportional to milk intake and the same is true amongst Seventh Day Adventists (Calcium and vitamin D, 1985). In Chicago, colon cancer incidence was found to vary inversely with the amount of calcium and vitamin D in the diet (Garland *et al.*, 1985). In studies by Lipkin and Newmark (1985) calcium was fed to patients considered to be at risk of developing colon cancer and its effect on the colonic mucosa monitored. Following calcium administration, the proliferative capacity of the colonic mucosa returned to the levels seen in individuals at low risk of developing colonic cancer. It was hypothesised that since calcium will bind the bile salts and free fatty acids characteristic of the Western diet within the lumen of the colon and render them insoluble, it protected the colon from the promoting effects of these compounds. Case-control studies from Japan, Norway, France and the Hawaiian Japanese have correlated increased sodium intake with increased mortality from cancer of the stomach and the colon (Tuyns, 1983). Schrauzer (1978) demonstrated that high zinc levels are associated with cancer of the colon.

Non-dietary factors

Non-dietary factors have not been a major consideration in the aetiology of colorectal carcinoma, mainly due to a lack of available evidence. Boyd and Doll (1954) showed that twice as many patients with gastro-intestinal cancers had used liquid paraffin regularly over the preceding 5 years, compared with a control group. However, liquid paraffin was known to contain fluorescent substances that could have been carcinogenic. No correlation between colorectal carcinoma and occupational exposure has been made although some data are available for the textile industry. Of five studies based on routinely collected cancer incidence or mortality data (Versluys, 1949; Guralnik, 1963; Delzell and Grufferman, 1983; Olsen and Jensen, 1987; Dubrow and Gute, 1988), one showed a significantly increased risk for colorectal cancer in spinners and weavers (Guralnik, 1963) and one found a significantly increased risk for rectal cancer, particularly in dyeing and finishing operations (Dubrow and Gute, 1988). Recently, a protective effect of early age at first pregnancy has been reported for colorectal carcinoma in women (Potter and McMichael, 1983; Howe *et al.*, 1985).

Overall conclusions

The aetiology of colorectal carcinoma is obviously complex and multifactorial. Few specific risk factors have been established other than genetic predisposition and diet. However, as adenomatous polyps are the precursors of colon carcinoma (Muto *et al.*, 1975; Chapter 1) and their geographic distribution and incidence in the population worldwide closely resembles that of elevated colon carcinoma risk, it is interesting to speculate that the development of sporadic adenomas is in large part genetically determined and that dietary factors are responsible for the malignant transformation (Schofield, 1982). The specific dietary factors have yet to be identified, but it is generally accepted that diets high in fat and cholesterol and low in cereal grains and fibre are associated with increased risk. Therefore, to quote from Cruse (1989), 'there are few comparable opportunities for preventing cancer so cheaply, safely and simply'.

References

Ames, B. N., McCann, J. and Yamasaki, E. (1975) Methods for detecting carcinogens and mutagens with the *Salmonella*/mammalian-microsome mutagenicity test. *Mutat. Res.*, **31**, 347–64.

Armstrong, B. and Doll, R. (1975) Environmental factors and cancer incidence and mortality in different countries with special reference to dietary practices. *Int. J. Cancer*, **15**, 617–31.

Askew, A. R., Ward, M., Green, M. K. and Reibelt, D. (1982) Faecal mutagenesis and colonic cancer. *Aust. N.Z. J. Surg.*, **52**, 27–9.

Bingham, S., Williams, D. R. H., Cole, T. J. and James, W. P. T. (1979) Dietary fibre and regional large-bowel cancer mortality in Britain. *Br. J. Cancer*, **40**, 456–63.

Bjelke, E. (1973) Epidemiologic studies of cancer of the stomach, colon and rectum, vols. 1–4. PhD thesis, University of Minnesota.

Bjelke, E. (1980) Epidemiology of colorectal cancer with emphasis on diet. In: *Human Cancer: Its Characterisation and Treatment*, pp. 158–74. Excerpta Medica, Amsterdam.

Blot, W. J., Fraumeni, J. F., Stone, B. J. and McKay, F. W. (1976) Geographic patterns of large bowel cancer in the US. *J. Natl. Cancer Inst.*, **57**, 1225–31.

Boyd, J. T. and Doll, R. (1954) Gastrointestinal cancer and the use of liquid paraffin. *Br. J. Cancer*, **8**, 231–7.

Bruce, W. R. and Dion, P. W. (1980) Studies relating to a faecal mutagen. *Am. J. Clin. Nutr.*, **33**, 2511–12.

Bruce, W. R., Varghese, A. J., Furrer, R. and Land, P. C. (1977) A mutagen in the faeces of normal humans. In: *Origins of Human Cancer*, ed. H. H. Hiatt, J. D. Watson and J. A. Winstein, pp. 1641–6. Cold Spring Harbor, New York.

Bruce, W. R., Baptista, J., Che, T., *et al.* (1982) General structure of fecapentaenes, the mutagenic substances in human faeces. *Naturwissenschaften*, **69**, 557–8.

Burkitt, D. P. (1971) Epidemiology of cancer of the colon and rectum. *Cancer*, **28**, 3–13.

Burkitt, D. P., Walker, A. R. P. and Painter, N. S. (1972) Effect of dietary fibre on stools and transit times and its role in the causation of disease. *Lancet*, **2**, 1408–12.

Calcium and vitamin D intakes influence the risk of bowel cancer in men (1985). *Nutr. Rev.*, **43**, 170–2.

Clark, L. C. (1985) The epidemiology of selenium and cancer. *Fed. Proc.*, **44**, 2584–9.

Committee on Diet, Nutrition and Cancer (1982) Assembly of Life Sciences, National Research Council. National Academy Press, Washington, DC.

Core, S. K. and Watne, A. L. (1974) Faecal steroids and colon cancer. *Fed. Proc.*, **33**, 260.

Correa, P. and Haenszel, W. (1978) The epidemiology of large-bowel cancer. *Adv. Cancer Res.*, **26**, 1–141.

Cruse, J. P. (1989) Cholesterol, neutral sterols and colorectal cancer. In: *Colorectal Cancer*, ed. H. K. Seitz, U. A. Simanowski and N. A. Wright, pp. 112–24. Springer, Berlin.

Cummings, J. H. (1985) Cancer of the large bowel. In: *Dietary Fibre, Fibre-Depleted Foods and Disease*, ed. H. Trowell *et al.*, pp. 161–9. Academic Press, London.

Dean, G., MacLennan, R., McLoughlin, H. and Shelley, E. (1979) Causes of death of blue-collar workers in a Dublin brewery 1954–1973. *Br. J. Cancer*, **40**, 581–9.

Delzell, E. and Grufferman, S. (1983) Cancer and other causes of death among female textile workers 1976–1978. *J. Natl. Cancer Inst.*, **71** 735–40.

Drasar, B. S. and Irving, D. (1973) Environmental factors and cancer of the colon and breast. *Br. J. Cancer*, **27**, 167–72.

Dubrow, R. and Gute, D. M. (1988) Cause-specific mortality among male textile workers in Rhode Island. *Am J. Ind. Med.*, **13**, 439–54.

Ehrich, M., Aswell, J. E., Van Tassell, R. H., *et al.* (1979) Mutagens in the faeces of 3 South African populations at different levels of risk for colon cancer. *Mutat. Res.*, **64**, 231–40.

Englyst, H. N. and Cummings, J. H., (1986) Measurement of dietary fibre as non-starch polysaccharides. In: *Dietary Fibre: Basic and Clinical Aspects*, ed. G. V. Vahouny and D. Kritchevsky, pp. 17–34. Plenum Press, New York.

Enstrom, J. E. (1977) Colorectal cancer and beer drinking. *Br. J. Cancer*, **35**, 647–83.

Faivre, J., Boutron, M. C., Hillon, P., *et al.* (1985) In: *Diet and Human Carcinogenesis*, ed. S. V. Joossens *et al.* pp. 123–36. Elsevier, Amsterdam.

Ferguson, L. R. and Alley, P. G. (1982) Faecal mutagens from population groups within New Zealand at different risk of colorectal cancer. In: *Mutagens in Our Environment*, ed. M. Sorba and M. Vaimo, pp. 423–9. A. R. Liss, New York.

Fraser, P. and Adelstein, A. M. (1982) Recent trends. In: *Colorectal Cancer*, ed. W. Duncan, pp. 1–10. Springer, Berlin.

Freeman, H. J. (1979) Dietary fibre and colonic neoplasia. *CMA J.* **121**, 291–6.

Garland, C., Barret-Connor, E., Rossof, A. H., *et al.* (1985) Dietary vitamin D and calcium and risk of colorectal cancer: a 19 year prospective study in men. *Lancet*, **9**, 307–9.

Goggleman, W., Maier, F. K. and Pfaendler, H. R. (1986) Mutagenicity of synthetic racemic fecapentaene-12. *Mutat. Res.*, **174**, 165–7.

Graham, S., Dayal, H., Swanson, M., Mittelmam, A. and Wilkinson, G. (1978) Diet in the epidemiology of cancer of the colon and rectum. *J. Natl. Cancer Inst.* **61**, 709–14.

Green, M. H. L. and Muriel, W. J. (1976) Mutagen testing using the TRP+ reversion in *E. coli. Mutat. Res.*, **38**, 3–32.

Green, M. H. L., Muriel, W. J. and Bridges, B. A. (1976) Use of a simplified fluctuation test to detect low levels of mutagens. *Mutat. Res.*, **38**, 33–42.

Greenwald, P., Korns, R. F., Nasca, P. C. and Wolfgang, P. E. (1975) Cancer in United States Jews. *Cancer Res.*, **35**, 3507–12.

Guralnik, L. (1963) *Mortality by Occupation and Cause of Death Among Men of 20–64 Years of Age, United States 1950*. Vital Statistics Special Reports 53, No. 3. Department of Health, Education and Welfare, Washington, DC.

Haenszel, W. (1961) Cancer mortality among the foreign-born in the United States. *J. Natl. Cancer Inst.*, **26**, 37–132.

Haenszel, W. (1971) Cancer mortality amongst US Jews. *Isr. J. Med. Sci.*, **7**, 1437–50.

Haenszel, W. (1982) Migrant studies. In: *Cancer Epidemiology and Prevention*, ed. D. Schottenfeld and J. F. Fraumeni, pp. 194–207. Saunders, Philadelphia.

Haenszel, W. and Dawson, E. A. (1965) A note on mortality from cancer of the colon and rectum in the United States. *Cancer*, **18**, 265–72.

Haenszel, W. and Kurihara, M. (1968) Studies of Japanese migrants. I. Mortality fron cancer and other diseases amongst Japanese in the United States. *J. Natl. Cancer Inst.*, **40**, 43–68.

Haenszel, W., Berg, J. W., Segi, M., *et al.* (1973) Large-bowel cancer in Hawaiian Japanese. *J. Natl. Cancer Inst.* **51**, 1765–79.

Haenszel, W., Locke, F. B. and Segi, M. (1980) A case-control study of large-bowel cancer in Japan. *J. Natl. Cancer Inst.*, **64**, 17–22.

Hayatsu, H., Hayatsu, T., Wataya, Y. and Mower, H. F. (1985) Faecal mutagenicity arising from ingestion of fried ground beef in the human. *Mutat. Res.*, **143**, 207–11.

Hill, M. J. (1974) Bacteria and the etiology of colonic cancer. *Cancer*, **34**, 815–18.

Hill, M. J. (1975) The role of colonic anaerobes in the metabolism of bile acids and steroids and its relation to colon cancer. *Cancer*, **36**, 2387–400.

Hill, M. J., Drasar, B. S., Aries, V., *et al.* (1971) Bacteria and the aetiology of cancer of the large bowel. *Lancet*, **1**, 95–100.

Hill, M. J., Morson, B. C. and Bussey, H. J. R. (1978) Etiology of the adenoma–carcinoma sequence in large bowel. Lancet, **1**, 245–7.

Hill, M. J., Morson B. C. and Thompson, M. H. (1983) The role of faecal bile acids (FBA) in large bowel carcinogenesis. *Br. J. Cancer*, **48**, 143.

Hirai, N., Kingston, D. G. I., Van Tassell, R. L. and Wilkins, T. D. (1982) Structure and elucidation of a potent mutagen from human faeces. *J. Am. Chem. Soc.*, **104**, 6149–50.

Howe, G. R., Craib, K. J. P. and Miller, A. B. (1985) Age at first pregnancy and risk of colorectal cancer. *J. Natl. Cancer Inst.*, **74**, 1155–9.

IARC, Intestinal Microecology Group (1977) Dietary fibre, transit time, faecal bacteria, steroids and colon cancer in 2 Scandinavian populations. *Lancet*, **2**, 207–11.

Isles, G. G., Hole, D. J., Gillis, C. R., *et al.* (1989) Plasma cholesterol, coronary heart disease and cancer in the Renfrew and Paisley study. *Br. Med. J.*, **298**, 920–4.

Jacobs, L. R. (1986*a*) Enhancement of experimental colon cancer and production of colitis in rats fed sorbital. *Clin. Res.*, **35**, 441A.

Jacobs, L. R. (1986*b*) Enhancement of experimental rat colon cancer with lactulose. *Gastroenterology*, **90**, 1473.

Jain, M., Cook, G. M., Davis, F. G., *et al.* (1980) A case-control study of diet and colorectal cancer. *Int. J. Cancer*, **26**, 757–68.

Jensen, O. M. (1979) Cancer morbidity and causes of death among Danish brewery workers. *Int. J. Cancer*, **23**, 454–63.

Jensen, O. M., MacLennan, B., Wahrendorf, J., *et al.* (1982) Diet, bowel function, faecal characterisation and large bowel cancer in Denmark and Finland. *Nutr. Cancer*, **4**, 5–19.

Kark, J. D., Smith, A. H. and Hames, C. G. (1980) The relationship of serum cholesterol to the incidence of cancer in Evans County, Georgia. *J. Chron. Dis.*, **33**, 311–22.

Kinlen, L. J. (1982*a*) Fat and cancer. In: *Aetiology in Colorectal Cancer*, ed. W. Duncan, pp. 11–20. Springer, Berlin.

Kinlen, L. J. (1982*b*) Meat and fat consumption and cancer mortality: a study of strict religious orders in Britain. *Lancet*, **1**, 946–9.

Kinlen, L. J. (1986) Fat and cancer aetiology. *Prog. Lipid Res.*, **25**, 527–31.

Knize, M. G., Andresen, B. D., Healy, S. K., *et al.* (1985) Effects of temperature, patty thickness and fat content on the production of mutagens in fried ground beef. *Food Chem. Toxicol.*, **23**, 1035–40.

Kuhnlein, H. V. and Kuhnlein, U. (1980) Mutagens in faeces from subjects on controlled formula diets. *Nutr. Cancer*, **2**, 119–24.

Kuhnlein, U., Bergstrom, D. and Kuhnlein, H. (1981) Mutagens in faeces from vegetarians and non-vegetarians. *Mutat. Res.*, **85**, 1–12.

Lanza, E. and Butrum, R. R. (1986) A critical review of food fibre analysis and data. *J. Am. Diet. Assoc.* **86**, 732–40.

Lee, H. P., Gourley, L., Duffy, S. W., *et al.* (1989) Colorectal cancer and diet in an Asian population: a case-control study among Singapore Chinese. *Int. J. Cancer*, **43**, 1007–16.

Lipkin, M. and Newmark, H. (1985) Effect of added dietary calcium on colonic epithelial cell proliferation in subjects at high-risk for familial colon cancer, *New. Engl. J. Med.*, **313**, 1381–4.

Liu, K., Moss, D., Persky, V., *et al.* (1979) Dietary cholesterol, fat and fibre in colon cancer mortality. *Lancet*, **2**, 782–5.

Lyon, J. L. and Sorenson, A. W. (1978) Colon Ca in low risk populations. *Am. J. Clin. Nutr.*, **31**, 5227–30.

McBurney, M. I., Van Soest, P. J. and Jeraci, J. L. (1987) Colonic carcinogenesis: the microbial feast or famine mechanisms. *Nutr. Cancer*, **10**, 23–8.

McDonald, I. A., Webb, G. R. and Mahony, D. E. (1978) Fecal hydroxysteroid dehydrogenase activities in Seventh-Day Adventists, control subjects and bowel cancer patients. *Am. J. Clin. Nutr.*, **31**, S233–8.

McMichael, A. J., Jensen, O.M., Parkin, D. M. and Zaridze, D. G. (1984) Dietary and endogenous cholesterol in human cancer. *Epidemiol. Rev.*, **6**, 192–216.

McMichael, A. J., McCall, M. G., Hartshorne, J. M. and Woodings, T. L. (1980) Patterns of gastrointestinal cancer in European migrants to Australia: the role of dietary change. *Int. J. Cancer*, **25**, 431–7.

Malhotra, S. L. (1967) Geographical distribution of intestinal cancers in India with special reference to causation. *Gut*, **8**, 361–72.

Mannes, G. A., Maier, A., Thieme, C., *et al.* (1986) Relationship between the frequency of colorectal adenoma and the serum cholesterol level. *New Engl. J. Med.*, **315**, 1634–8.

Manousos, O., Day, N. E., Trichopoulos, D., *et al.* (1983) Diet and colorectal cancer: a case-control study in Greece. *Int. J. Cancer*, **32**, 1–5.

Maron, D. M. and Ames, B. N. (1983) Revised methods for the *Salmonella* mutagenicity test. *Mutat. Res.*, **113**, 173–215.

Modan, B., Barell, V., Lubin, F., Modan, M. and Greenberg, R. A. (1975) Low-fibre intake as an etiologic factor in cancer of the colon. *J. Natl. Cancer Inst.*, **55**, 15–18.

Moore, W. E. C. and Holdeman, L. V. (1974) Human faecal flora: the normal flora of 20 Japanese Hawaiians *Appl. Microbiol.*, **27**, 961–79.

Moore, W. E. C., Cato, E. P. and Holdeman, L. V. (1978) Some clinical concepts in intestinal bacteriology. *Am. J. Clin. Nutr.*, **31**, 533–542.

Monk, M. and Warshauer, M. E. (1975) Stomach and colon cancer mortality among Puerto Ricans in New York City and Puerto Rico. *J. Anatomic. Dis.*, **28**, 349–58.

Mower, H. F., Ichinosubo, D., Wang, L. W. *et al.* (1982) Faecal mutagens in two Japanese populations with different colon cancer risks. *Cancer Res.*, **42**, 1164–9.

Muto, T., Bussey, H. J. R. and Morson, B. C. (1975) The evolution of cancer of the colon and rectum. *Cancer*, **36**, 2251–70.

Nagao, M., Wakabayashi, K. and Sugimura, T. (1985) Mutagens in food and drinks and their carcinogenicity. In: *Mutagenicity Testing in Environmental Pollution Control*, ed. F. K. Zimmerman and R. E. Taylor-Mayer, pp. 69–85. Ellis Horwood, Chichester.

Nelson, R. (1987) Dietary minerals and colon carcinogenesis. *Anticancer Res.*, **7**, 259–70.

Newill, V. A. (1961) Distribution of cancer mortality among ethnic subgroups of the white population of New York City 1953–1958. *J. Natl. Cancer Inst.*, **26**, 405–17.

Nilsson, L., Overik, E., Fredholm, L., *et al.* (1986) Influence of frying fat on mutagenic activity in lean pork meat. *Mutat. Res.*, **171**, 115–21.

Olsen, J. H. and Jensen, O. M. (1987) Occupation and risk of cancer in Denmark. *Scand. J. Work Environ. Health*, **13** (Suppl.), 1–19.

Overik, E., Nilsson, L., Fredholm, L., *et al.* (1984) High mutagenic activity formed in pan-broiled pork. *Mutat. Res.*, **135**, 149–57.

Peto, R., Doll, R., Buckely, J. D. and Sporn, M. B. (1981) Can dietary ß-carotene materially reduce human cancer rates? *Nature*, **29**, 201–8.

Phillips, R. L. and Snowdon, D. A. (1983) Association of meat and coffee use with cancers of the large bowel, breast and prostate among Seventh-Day Adventists: preliminary results. *Cancer Res.*, (Suppl.) **43**, 24035–85.

Phillips, R. L., Garfinkel, L., Kuzma, J. W., Beeson, W. L., Lotz, T. and Brin, B. (1980) Mortality amongst Californian Seventh Day Adventists for selected cancer sites. *J. Natl. Cancer Inst.*, **65**, 1097–107.

Pietroiusti, A., Giuliano, M., Vita, S., *et al.* (1983) Fecal pH and cancer of the large bowel. *Gastroenterology*, **84**, 1273.

Plummer, S. M., Graftstrom, R. C., Yang, L. L., *et al.* (1986) Fecapentaene-12 causes DNA damage and mutation in human cells. *Carcinogenesis*, **7**, 1607–9.

Potter, J. D. and McMichael, A. J. (1983) Large-bowel cancer in women in relation to reproductive and hormonal factors: a case-control study. *J. Natl., Cancer Inst.*, **71**, 703–9.

Reddy, B. S. (1980) Dietary fibre and colon cancer: epidemiologic and experimental evidence. *CMA J.*, **123**, 850–6.

Reddy, B. S. (1986) Faecal mutagens as a function of diet. *Prog. Clin. Biol. Res.*, **206**, 213–24.

Reddy, B. S. and Wynder, E. L. (1973) Large bowel carcinogenesis: faecal constitutents of populations with diverse incidence rates of colon cancer. *J. Natl. Cancer Inst.*, **50**, 1437–42.

Reddy, B. S. and Wynder. E. L. (1977) Metabolic epidemiology of colon cancer: faecal bile acids and neutral sterols in colon cancer patients and patients with adenomatous polyps. *Cancer*, **39**, 2533–9.

Reddy, B. S., Mastromarino, A., Gustafson, C., *et al.* (1976) Faecal bile acids and neutral sterols in patients with familial polyposis. *Cancer*, **38**, 1694–8.

Reddy, B. S., Hedges, A. R., Loakso, K., *et al.* (1978) Metabolic epidemiology of large bowel cancer: faecal bulk and consistency of high-risk North American and low-risk Finnish population. *Cancer*, **42**, 2832–48.

Reddy, B. S., Sharma, C., Darby, L., *et al.* (1980*a*) Metabolic epidemiology of large-bowel cancer: faecal mutagens in high- and low-risk populations for colon cancer. *Mutat. Res.*, **72**, 511–22.

Reddy, B. S., Sharma, C. and Wynder, E. L. (1980*b*) Faecal factors which might modify the formula of faecal co-mutagens in high and low-risk populations for colon cancer. *Cancer Lett.*, **10**, 123–32.

Reddy, B. S., Sharma, C., Matthews L., *et al.* (1985) Metabolic epidemiology of colon cancer: faecal mutagenesis in healthy subjects from rural Kuopia and urban Helsinki, Finland. *Mutat. Res.*, **152**, 97–105.

Rose. G. and Shipley, M. J. (1980) Plasma lipids and mortality: a source of error. *Lancet*, **1**, 523–6.

Salyers, A. A., Palmer, J. K. and Wilkins, T. D. (1977) Laminarase (ß-glucanase) activity in *Bacteroides* from the human colon. *Appl. Env. Microbiol.*, **33**, 1118–24.

Samelson, S. L., Nelson, R. L. and Nyhus, L. M. (1985) Protective role of faecal pH in experimental colon carcinogenesis. *J. R. Soc. Med.*, **78**, 208–33.

Schatzkin, A., Hoover, R. N., Taylor, P. R., *et al.* (1987) Serum cholesterol and cancer in the NHANES 1 epidemiologic follow-up study. *Lancet*, **2**, 298–301.

Schofield, P. F. (1982) Carcinoma of the rectum. In: *Surgical Review 3*, ed. J. S. P. Lumley and J. L. Craven, pp. 178–207. Pitman, Bath.

Schrauzer, G. N. (1978) Trace elements, nutrition and cancer: perspectives of prevention. In: *Inorganic and Nutritional Aspects of Cancer*, pp. 323–44. Plenum Press, New York.

Seidman, H. (1970) Cancer deaths by site and sex for religious and socioeconomic groups in New York City. *Environ. Res.*, **3**, 234–50.

Seidman, H. (1971) Cancer mortality in New York City for country of birth, religious and socioeconomic groups. *Environ, Res.*, **4**, 390–429.

Sian, M. S. (1987) Diet and nutritional factors in the aetiology of colon cancer (review). *Anticancer Res.*, **7**, 293–300.

Slattery, M. L., Sorenson, A. W., Mahoney, A. W., *et al.* (1988) Diet and colon cancer: assessment of risk by fiber type and food source. *J. Natl. Cancer Inst.*, **80**, 1474–80.

Smith, R.L. (1956) Recorded and expected mortality among the Japanese of the United States and Hawaii with special reference to cancer. *J. Natl. Cancer Inst.*, **17**, 459–73.

Sorlie, P. D. and Feinlieb, M. (1982) The serum cholesterol–cancer relationship: an analysis of time-trends in the Framlingham study, *J. Natl. Cancer Inst.*, **69**, 989–96.

Stemmerman, G. N., Nomura, A. M. Y. and Heilbrun, L. K. (1984) Dietary fat and risk of colorectal cancer. *Cancer Res.*, **44**, 4633–7.

Stocks, P. (1958) Cancer incidence in North Wales and Liverpool region in relation to habits and environment. Cancer Campaign London, 35th Annual Report.

Strobel, H. W. and Fang, W. F. (1981) Role of cytochrome p-450 in the response of the colon to xenobiotics. In: *Banbury Report 7*, ed. W. R. Bruce *et al.* pp. 141–9. Cold Spring Harbor, New York.

Sugimura, T. (1985) Carcinogenicity of mutagenic heterocyclic amines formed during the cooking process. *Mutat. Res.*, **150**, 33–41.

Tornberg, S. A. Holm, L.-E., Cartensen, J. *et al.* (1986) Risks of cancer of the colon and rectum in relation to serum cholesterol and beta-lipoprotein. *New Engl. J. Med.*, **315**, 1629–33.

Tuyns, A. J. (1983) Sodium chloride and cancer of the digestive tract. *Nutr. Cancer*, **4**, 198–205.

Van Tassell, R. L., MacDonald, D. K. and Wilkins, T. D. (1982*a*) Stimulation of mutagen production in human faeces by bile and bile acids. *Mutat. Res.*, **103**, 233–9.

Van Tassell, R. L., MacDonald, D. K. and Wilkins, T. D. (1982*b*) Production of a faecal mutagen by *Bacteroides* ssp. *Infect. Immunol.*, **37**, 975–80.

Venitt, S. (1981) Faecal mutagens: their discovery and possible relevance to the aetiology of large-bowel cancer in man. In: *Progress in Mutation Research*, ed. A. Kappas, vol. 2, pp. 3–10. Elsevier/North-Holland Biomedical Press, Amsterdam.

Venitt, S. (1982) Mutagens in human faeces: are they relevant to cancer of the large bowel? *Mutat. Res.*, **98**, 265–86.

Venitt, S. (1988) Mutagens in human faeces and cancer of the large bowel. In: *Role of the Gut Flora in Toxicity and Cancer*, pp. 399–460. Academic Press, New York.

Venitt, S., Bosworth, D. and Alldrick, A. J. (1986) Pilot study of the effect of diet on the mutagenicity on human faeces. *Mutagenesis*, **1**, 353–8.

Venitt, S., Bosworth, D. and Easton, D. F. (1987) Lack of mutagenic activity of bile acids in bacterial fluctuation tests. *Mutat. Res.*, **190**, 191–6.

Versluys, J. J. (1949) Cancer and occupation in the Netherlands. *Br. J. Cancer*, **3**, 161–85.

Walker, A. R. P., Walker, B. F. and Walker, A. J. (1986) Faecal pH, dietary fibre intake and proneness to colon cancer in four South African populations. *Br. J. Cancer*, **53**, 489–95.

Watabe, J. and Bernstein, H. (1985) The mutagenicity of bile acids using a fluctuation test. *Mutat. Res.*, **158**, 45–51.

Waterhouse, J., Shanmugaratnam, K., Mair, C. and Powell, J. (eds.) (1982) *Cancer Incidence in Five Continents*, vol. IV. IARC Scientific Publication No. 42. Lyon, France.

Wilkins, T. D., Lederman, M., Van Tassell, R. L. *et al.* (1980) Characterisation of a mutagenic bacterial product in human faeces. *Am. J. Clin. Nutr.*, **33**, 2513–20.

Wilkins, T. D. and Van Tassell, R. L. (1983) Bacterial mutagens in human colon. In: *Human Intestinal Microflora in Health and Disease*, ed. D. J. Hentges, pp. 265–88. Academic Press, New York.

Wynder, E. L. (1987) Amount and type of fat/fiber in nutritional carcinogenesis. *Prev. Med.*, **16**, 451–9.

Wynder, E. L. and Reddy, B. S. (1978) In: *Colon Cancer. Cancer Campaign* vol. 2, ed. E. Grindman, pp. 1–4. Fischer-Verlag, Stuttgart.

Wynder, E. and Shigematsu, T. (1967) Environmental factors of cases of the colon and rectum. *Cancer*, **20**, 1520–61.

Zaridze, D. G. (1983) Environmental aetiology of large-bowel cancer. *J. Natl. Cancer Inst.*, **70**, 389–400.

Zhang, Y. Q., MacLennan, R. and Berry, G. (1984) Mortality of Chinese in New South Wales 1969–1978. *Int. J. Epidemiol.* **13**, 188–92.

Ziegler, R. G., Devesa, S. S. and Fraumeni, J. F. (1986) Epidemiologic patterns of colorectal cancer. *Imp. Adv. Oncol.*, **1**, 209–32.

4

In vivo experimental models

The evidence presented so far in this book suggests that genetic variation accounts for only a small proportion of human colorectal carcinomas (Chapter 2) and that environmental factors, most probably dietary (Chapter 3), are important and causal in the great majority of cases. Although the carcinogens responsible for human colorectal carcinoma are still not known (Bruce, 1986, 1987), animal models can be used to evaluate the risk factors and protective factors identified by the epidemiologists and provide an insight into their mechanisms of action. One thing that is certain is that the presence of the faecal stream is essential for the promotion of colorectal tumours in the animal model. Studies in which part of the gut was isolated by surgical intervention (Williamson *et al.*, 1980) showed that the rate of tumour formation in the isolated section was always much lower than in those portions of the gut with a normal faecal stream.

The rodent as a model for human colorectal cancer

Rats and mice treated with 1,2-dimethylhydrazine (DMH) or with one of its metabolites azoxymethane (AOM) or methyl azoxymethanol acetate (MAM) are the most widely used models for large bowel cancer (Ward *et al.*, 1973; Weisburger and Fiala 1983). DMH and AOM are procarcinogens with a high degree of specificity for the intestinal mucosa. It is known that they are metabolised in the liver by pathways that include alcohol dehydrogenase and the mixed function oxidases and that MAM, the hepatic metabolite of DMH, and AOM reach the colon via the blood stream rather than the bile. The adenocarcinomas produced are histologically similar to human colon tumours (Shamsuddin, 1983; Teague, 1983; Nakamura and Kino, 1985) but are more frequently polypoid and less frequently deeply invasive than human tumours. There are, however, two major dissimilarities between the experimental and human situations. First of all, in AOM-treated rats microglandular adenocarcinomas with extracellular mucin occur commonly in the lymphoid nodules of the ascending colon, caecum and descending colon. This type of carcinoma is rare in humans. Secondly, rodent liver is resistant to metastases, whilst hepatic metastases are common in the human situation.

Experimentally induced adenomas and carcinomas have both been identified, but whether progression from benign to malignant lesions occurs is less clear (Madara *et al.*, 1983). Maskens and Dujardin-Loits (1981) concluded that adenomas were found in mice, but only rarely in rats. Many malignant animal tumours gave no evidence of originating from benign tumours and even in studies in which the animals were examined at several stages, the evidence for progression was not strong (Maskens and Dujardin-Loits, 1981; Shamsuddin, 1983). In experimental animals malignant tumours were found as early if not earlier than adenomas, but the high doses of carcinogen used in most studies may have precluded the observation of the adenoma–carcinoma sequence that is so characteristic of tumour development in humans. What is certain is that the immediate precursor of a grossly visible tumour in an animal is the appearance of a microscopic focus of epithelial dysplasia in an otherwise normal colonic crypt (Hamilton *et al.*, 1982). Abnormal epithelial proliferation can be found throughout the colon (Lipkin, 1983; Tutton and Barkla, 1983) and is associated with changes in ornithine decarboxylase activity (ODC) and prostaglandin production. Inhibitors of both ODC activity and prostaglandin biosynthesis have been shown to reduce carcinogen-induced colon tumourigenesis in rats (see later).

Chemical induction of colon cancer

DMH is activated via azomethane, AOM and MAM to yield the ultimate carcinogen (Weisburger and Fiala, 1983). Both AOM and MAM are specific colon carcinogens in rodents (Ward *et al.*, 1973; Weisburger and Fiala, 1983) and more effective than DMH on a molar basis. DMH metabolism varies with dose and route of administration (Druckrey *et al.*, 1967; Toth and Patil, 1982).

The first step in DMH-induced colon carcinogenesis appears to be alkylation of the target organ (Maskens, 1980). Both *N*-7-methylguanine (7-MeG) and *O*-6-methylguanine (O^6MeG) have been isolated from the colonic mucosal DNA of rats treated with ^{14}C-labelled DMH (Hawks and Magee, 1974; Rogers and Pegg, 1977; Swenberg *et al.*, 1979) and from cultured rat colon after incubation with labelled DMH (Autrup and Williams, 1983). Compounds that inhibit DMH metabolism (e.g. disulfiram and pyrazole) decrease O^{6}MeG formation in rat colonic DNA. Generally speaking the extent of colonic DNA alkylation in rats and mice is proportional to the susceptibility to DMH-induced colon carcinogenesis (Cooper *et al.*, 1978; Pollard and Luckert, 1980). Serial administration of DMH causes an expansion of the proliferative zone and the cell proliferation activity of the colonic crypts (Heitman *et al.*, 1983; Deschner and Maskens, 1983; Wright and Alison, 1984; Deschner, 1985; Jacobs and Lupton, 1986). DMH is known to increase crypt column height and hyperplasia and hypertrophy of the colonic crypt epithelium. It is known from several studies in both animals and humans that cell proliferation during the initiation phase of carcinogenesis leads to enhanced tumourigenesis (Jacobs, 1983, 1984; Farber, 1984; Romagnoli *et al.*, 1984; Williamson and Rainey, 1984).

Other large bowel carcinogens that have been used include benzo[*a*]-pyrene and dimethylbenzanthracene (DMBA), and the direct-acting carcinogens *N*-methyl-*N′*-nitro-*N*-nitrosoguanidine (MNNG) and *N*-methyl-*N*-nitrosourea (MNU), all of which induce tumours at the site of application in the colon and rectum (Narisawa and Weisburger, 1975; Narisawa *et al.*, 1981). Certainly intrarectal administration of either MNU or MNNG results in the induction of adenomas, adenocarcinomas, sarcomas and hyperplastic polyps, depending on the dose and species of animal used (Ward *et al.*, 1973; Nauss *et al.*, 1984*b*). Low dose MNU-induced neoplasms have really been quite effective in the study of the modifying effects of certain environmental factors on colon carcinogenesis.

There are, however, several important points to be emphasised about such studies. The dose of carcinogen affects the latent period and the characteristics of tumourigenesis. Higher doses generally lead to shorter latent periods, higher tumour incidence and prevalence and greater multiplicity. Inappropriately high or low doses may preclude detecting the effects of modulating agents. The route of administration and the animals used can affect the organ specificity of some carcinogens. Carcinogens that require activation might induce tumours at sites other than the colon, whereas direct-acting carcinogens induce tumours at the site of application in the colon. Even within species, different strains of mice exhibit different susceptibilities with the same experimental protocol (Weisburger and Fiala, 1983; Glickman *et al.*, 1987). For all rodents, males and younger animals are more susceptible. Diets are also a critical consideration in the chemical induction of colon cancer, because dietary components are usually the modulatory agents being studied. Careful attention has to be paid to the individual nutrients and to the level of dietary

Table 4.1. *Criteria to be fulfilled by putative dietary carcinogens in animal studies (Cruse, 1989)*

1. Irrespective of the animal model used, the feeding of a diet containing the putative co-carcinogen should significantly augment the development, growth or spread of large bowel cancer
2. Diets completely lacking the co-carcinogen should show significant protective effects (increased latent period and survival or reduced incidence, multiplicity or size of large bowel tumours)
3. A dose–response relationship should be demonstrable between dietary intake of the co-carcinogen and the effect
4. A biochemically testable mechanism of co-carcinogenic action should be postulated, tested and demonstrated
5. The physiological conditions for co-carcinogenesis should be present in the animals
6. The biochemical levels of the putative co-carcinogen should be significantly different in the body fluids of the carcinogen-treated animals fed the co-carcinogen compared with the controls
7. The removal, inhibition or reduction of the co-carcinogen in the diet should be associated with a corresponding reduction in the co-carcinogenic effect

consumption (Reddy *et al.*, 1987). Thus, an unpalatable compound has the potential to reduce tumourigenesis by reducing the dietary intake, rather than by the direct effects of the compound itself. Tumourigenesis is the end-point of a complex series of events and irrespective of the carcinogen used is susceptible to dietary modification (LaMont and O'Gorman, 1978). As a consequence, the criteria that have to be fulfilled by putative dietary carcinogens in dietary studies must be carefully outlined (Cruse, 1989; Table 4.1).

Influence of dietary factors on colonic cancer in rodents

Dietary fat

Animal models in which dietary factors are controlled have provided a useful adjunct to epidemiological studies. Colon tumourigenesis induced by DMH, AOM, MAM, MNU and DMBA has been shown to be enhanced by high-fat diets (reviewed Newberne and Sahaphong, 1989). To date approximately thirty different trials from nine major laboratories have examined the influence of dietary fat on colon cancer in rodents.

One of the many criticisms of what should have been useful early studies was that the fat was simply added to the normal laboratory 'chow' or to purified diets, with the result that the diets were not isocalorifically balanced (Reddy *et al.*, 1977*a*, *b*; Bansal *et al.*, 1978; Bull *et al.*, 1979). This was important because, as we now know, there is decreased nutrient consumption in animals fed high-fat diets that are not nutritionally balanced. These nutritional imbalances rather than the level of dietary fat might therefore have had a significant influence on colon carcinogenesis.

A review of the data (Newberne and Sahaphong, 1989) showed that increased dietary fat had a positive effect in many, but not all of the studies, increasing either the incidence or number of tumours per animal (Table 4.2). Nigro *et al.* (1975) demonstrated that when beef tallow was added to the laboratory animal 'chow' of AOM-treated rats the number of intestinal tumours was increased. However, since the carcinogen dose was high, all the treated animals developed tumours. Multiple tumours were produced per animal and a 114 per cent increase in small intestinal tumours and a 48 per cent increase in colon tumours was observed. Reddy *et al.* (1976*a*) and Reddy and Ohmori (1981) reported that carcinogen-treated Fischer rats fed 20 per cent lard, 20 per cent corn oil or 20 per cent beef fat, had a higher incidence of adenomas than rats fed 5 per cent levels of the same fats. There were no differences among the diet groups in the incidence of adenocarcinomas. However, many of the better controlled later studies (Locniskar *et al.*, 1983; Nauss *et al.*, 1983, 1984*a*, *b*) have failed to support the hypothesis that dietary fat alone influences colon cancer, and suggest that there are other factors that might interact with fat to enhance tumour incidence.

Caloric intake, for example, appears to have a significant effect on the risk of tumours as reported by Visek and Clinton (1983) for breast cancer. Therefore, diets which differ in calories and which modify food intake must be taken into consideration. A study (Newberne and Sahaphong, 1989) of the effect of DMH on colon tumour incidence in Sprague–Dawley (SD) rats versus Fischer 344 (F344) rats, showed that F344 rats to be more sensitive to the toxic effects of DMH and that the deficit in weight gain was greatest for the animals fed the non-isocalorically balanced diet with the lowest concentration of certain vitamins and minerals. For the SD group the tumour incidence was 57 per cent in the group fed 20 per cent fat versus 27–33 per cent in the other three diet groups. Dietary treatment had no significant effect on colon tumour incidence or frequency (number of tumours per tumour-bearing animal) in F344 rats. However, a caloric intake comparison in SD versus F344 rats showed that the tumour incidence in the SD rats could be related to caloric intake. The SD and F344 rats differed significantly in their rate of weight gain and final body mass and an interesting aspect of the data was that the 1-month intake data prior to carcinogen treatment showed that the SD rats which were eating more prior to DMH carcinogen treatment were more likely to develop tumours.

Both human and animal studies have shown that the consumption of high-fibre diets is associated with increased faecal fat loss and therefore a reduced availability of calories (Nyman and Asp, 1982; Cummings, 1983; Isaksson *et al.*, 1984; Kaur *et al.*, 1985; Nauss *et al.*, 1987). One could postulate, therefore, that increased caloric intake could modify human or animal metabolism early in life to increase the risk later. In support of this, are the facts that men consume more fat and calories early on in their lives than women and that their colon cancer death rate is correspondingly higher. This is particularly evident in the black population of the USA. Also, with reference to the rat strain effect cited above, the more rapidly growing SD rat with the higher caloric intake was at a greater risk of tumour development and studies in which the caloric intake was increased immediately after birth by artificially reducing the litter size showed the increased caloric intake to increase the DMH-induced tumour risk (Newberne and Sahaphong, 1989).

Dietary cholesterol

The epidemiological data available to date neither refute nor support the conclusion that cholesterol-rich diets have a causal relationship to colorectal cancer (Lilienfeld, 1981; Committee on Nutrition, Diet and Cancer, 1982; McMichael *et al.*, 1984; Broitman, 1986). Liu *et al.* (1979) found a highly significant correlation between colon cancer mortality and cholesterol-rich diets in twenty industrialised countries, whilst a Canadian study (Jain *et al.*, 1980) showed a significant risk of colorectal cancer associated with increasing cholesterol intake, which was dose related.

Human studies, as stated previously, rarely produce clear-cut answers to questions linking diet and cancer, because they are retrospective and human recall is poor. Animal studies on the other hand, if designed properly, should be able to identify a cause and effect relationship. Rodent models in spite of the use of different carcinogens, different strains of rats and different diets, suggest that cholesterol is a potent dietary co-carcinogen or promoter (Broitman *et al.*, 1977; Cruse *et al.*, 1978*a*; Hiramatsu *et al.*, 1983; Klurfeld *et al.*, 1983). Cholesterol alone is not carcinogenic (Cruse *et al.*, 1978*a*).

Patients with colon cancer are known to have high levels of faecal cholesterol (Reddy and Wynder, 1977) as are patients with diseases known to be associated with or predisposing to colon cancer, such as FPC (FAP) (Reddy *et al.*, 1976*b*), Gardner's syndrome (Core and Watne, 1974) and ulcerative colitis (Reddy *et al.*, 1977*c*). Cholesterol enters the lumen of the large bowel by several routes including bile and exfoliated intestinal

Table 4.2. *The effect of dietary fat on colon tumourigenesis (Newberne and Sahaphong, 1989)*

Animal	Diet	Effect of high-fat diet on colon tumourigenesis	Reference
No carcinogen			
F7BL/1	0% vs. 10% added corn oil[a]	Increased incidence	El-Khatib and Cora (1981)
DMH			
Male and female Fischer rat	5% vs. 20% corn oil or lard[b]	Increased incidence and frequency of tumours	Reddy *et al.* (1977*a, b*)
Male Sprague–Dawley rat	5% vs. 20% coconut oil[b]	Increased frequency	Broitman *et al.* (1977)
Male Fischer rat	5% vs. 20% beef fat[b]	Increased incidence and frequency of colon adenomas	Reddy *et al.* (1977*a, b*)
Male W/Fu rat	5% vs. 30% corn oil[b]	Increased incidence and metastasis; decreased latency time	Bansal *et al.* (1978)
Male Sprague–Dawley rat	15% corn oil vs. 30% beef fat	Increased cumulative probability of death	Rogers *et al.* (1980)
Male Sprague–Dawley rat	5% mixed fat vs. 24% corn oil or 24% beef fat or 24% Crisco[c]	None	Nauss *et al.* (1984*a,b*), Newberne and Nauss (1986)
Male BALB/c mouse	5% mixed fat vs. 30% mixed fat[d]	None	Nutter *et al.* (1983)
Male Sprague–Dawley rat	5% corn oil vs. 24% corn oil[c]	None	Nauss *et al.* (1987)
ACM			
Male Sprague–Dawley rat	5% vs. 30% beef fat[b]	Increased frequency	Bull *et al.* (1979)
Male Sprague–Dawley rat	Low fat vs. 35% beef fat[a]	Increased frequency and incidence	Nigro *et al.* (1975)
MAM			
Male Fischer rat	5% vs. 20% beef fat[a]	Increased incidence and frequency of adenomas	Reddy *et al.* (1977*a, b*)
MNU			
Male Fischer rat	5% vs. 20% beef fat[b]	Increased incidence and frequency of adenomas	Reddy *et al.* (1977*a, b*)
Male Sprague–Dawley rat	5% mixed fat vs. 24% corn oil or 24% beef fat or 24% Crisco[c]	None	Nauss *et al.* (1984*a*)

Table 4.2 (*cont.*)

Animal	Diet	Effect of high-fat diet on colon tumourigenesis	Reference
3,2-Dimethyl-4-aminobiphenyl			
Male Fischer rat	5% vs. 23% beef fat[c]	Increased incidence and frequency in conventional but not germ-free rats	Reddy and Ohmori (1981)

Notes: Types of diets: [a]natural product; [b]semipurified, non-isocaloric; [c]semipurified, isocaloric; [d]mixed semipurified and natural product.

epithelial cells. As it is poorly absorbed, any excess cholesterol is excreted via the colon. Therefore the colonic epithelial cells of individuals on cholesterol-rich diets are exposed to high levels of faecal cholesterol and the metabolites of bacterial degradation, the neutral sterols coprostanone and coprostanol. Cholesterol-fed rats show a 20-fold greater excretion of neutral sterols than animals fed control diets (Hiramatsu *et al.*, 1983). Increased neutral sterol excretion was also correlated in some studies with carcinogen treatment (Reddy *et al.*, 1974*b*). Studies of cholesterol degradation by Hiramatsu *et al.* (1983) showed that cholesterol-fed rats had a lower conversion rate than those on the control diet. Since cholesterol feeding of carcinogen-treated animals significantly increased their colon cancer risk, the results suggest that the increased excretion of unchanged faecal cholesterol may be more harmful than an excess of cholesterol metabolites. A similar low conversion pattern is observed in individuals with FPC (FAP). However, it is probably worth noting that direct intrarectal administration of either cholesterol or its metabolites to rats treated with the direct-acting carcinogen MNNG failed to produce any co-carcinogenic effect (Reddy and Watanabe, 1979). This suggests that ingestion is the correct route for co-carcinogenic activity and suggests an additional requirement for the correct physiological conditions within the lumen.

The situation regarding serum cholesterol is even less clear, as alluded to earlier in Chapter 3 for human studies. In one animal study (Broitman *et al.*, 1977), DMH-treated rats fed cholesterol-rich diets together with saturated fats to enhance absorption, developed increased serum cholesterol levels but reduced colon cancer when compared with rats fed cholesterol-rich diets with polyunsaturated fats to inhibit cholesterol absorption. Three other experiments, however, showed increased serum cholesterol levels associated with cholesterol-induced co-carcinogenesis

(Hiramatsu *et al.*, 1983; Klurfield *et al.*, 1983; Barton *et al.*, 1987). Taken together, therefore, the human and experimental evidence strongly suggests a role for cholesterol in colon carcinoma, which may be synergistic with other dietary components.

Bile acids

Three bile acids predominate in human bile: cholic acid, chenodeoxycholic acid and deoxycholic acid. The most abundant bile acids in faeces are lithocholic and deoxycholic acids resulting from the bacterial degradation of chenodeoxycholic and cholic acid respectively. In addition, bile acids can undergo other modifications to produce a wide spectrum of minor faecal bile acids. Healthy humans excrete 500–750 mg of bile acids daily (Hofmann, 1977) and these amounts have been reported to increase in individuals with intestinal diseases (Reddy *et al.*, 1976*b*; Mastromarino *et al.*, 1978; Moskovitz *et al.*, 1979; Mudd *et al.*, 1980; Hill *et al.*, 1983) and increased risk of developing colon cancer (Reddy *et al.*, 1976*b*, 1977*b*, 1980; Reddy and Wynder, 1977).

Once again animal models provided the opportunity for a controlled study of the possible causal role of bile acids in colon carcinogenesis. Cholesterol is the obligatory precursor of bile acids, whilst high-fat diets increase bile output. Narisawa *et al.* (1974) were amongst the very first to provide evidence that bile acids might act as tumour promoters in animals following MNNG treatment, and Reddy and Watanabe (1979) showed lithocholic acid to increase adenocarcinomas. Previously, Nigro *et al.* (1973) had shown cholestyramine, a non-absorbable ion exchange resin with a strong affinity for bile salts, to enhance DMH- and AOM-induced tumours in rats. It was assumed that this was because the loss of the bile salts as a result of the cholestyramine was compensated for by bile acid synthesis in the liver resulting in an overall increase in bile salts. Bile acids administered intrarectally in the absence of carcinogen were not carcinogenic. Similar tumour enhancement was observed when cholic and chenodeoxycholic acids were administered in the diet following MNU treatment (Sarwal *et al.*, 1979; Cohen *et al.*, 1980). Thus, bile acids are active promoters whether administered intrarectally or in the diet. In some studies, however, differences were seen for specific bile acids depending on the route of administration, which suggested that not only the structure of the bile acids was important for their physiological action but also their interaction with the intestinal microflora and intestinal environment. Interestingly, a recent study (Tanida *et al.*, 1989) on the effects of the administration of sulpholithocholic acid and lithocholic acid salts showed that sulpholithocholic acid, which was not expected to be harmful, promoted colon carcinogenesis in F344 rats treated with MNU. Sulphation is considered to be one of the defence mechanisms which facilitates faster elimination of lithocholic acid from the body. However, in this case it was suggested that sulphation acted as the vehicle which allowed the lithocholic acid to be carried into the large intestine where it could act directly, avoiding absorption by the intestines. Further support for the role of bile acids in colon carcinogenesis is provided by studies on AOM-treated rats in which surgically diverting the bile ducts to the middle portion of the intestine resulted in an increase in colonic neoplasms.

However, it is clear that the causative role for bile acids in colon cancer does not occur in isolation from other dietary factors. For instance the quantity of fat ingested seems to determine the amounts of bile acids reaching the intestine, as does the composition of the intestinal microflora responsible for the degradation of bile acids. Dietary fibre may act by increasing faecal bulk and diluting potential carcinogens or promoters.

Dietary fibre

Epidemiological studies (Chapter 3) suggest a protective effect for fibre-containing foods on colorectal cancer. However, the only controlled prospective studies on dietary fibre and colon cancer have been done in animals. Also, animal studies using defined fibre sources have allowed the analysis of the roles played by different types of fibre in modulating the colorectal cancer risk.

Wheat bran is the most widely studied fibre supplement (Table 4.3). In mice two out of three experiments showed tumour enhancement (Clapp *et al.*, 1984), whilst in rats the majority of the experiments showed fibre to confer a protective effect on DMH- and AOM-treated animals. However, no protective effect of wheat bran was observed in rats following treatment with the direct-acting carcinogen MNU; protection was observed following treatment with MNNG, but only when fat intake was high (Kroes *et al.*, 1986).

Interestingly, other forms of bran did not exhibit the same protective effect under the same conditions. A comparison of the mechanisms whereby some brans protect against tumourigenesis whilst others enhance it was made by Clapp *et al.* (1984). They found a positive correlation between tumour incidence and the percentage of neutral detergent fibre in the bran. Wheat bran was shown to stimulate colonic epithelial cell growth, and presumably enhance tumour development, when fed only during the period of carcinogenic exposure. The same wheat bran supplement was shown to inhibit carcinogenesis when administered after carcinogen exposure (Jacobs, 1983). Tumour enhancement for oat bran

Table 4.3. *Dietary wheat bran and experimental colon cancer (summarised from Jacobs 1989)*

Carcinogen	Animal	Strain	Sex	Bran[a] (%)	Effect[b]	Reference
DMH	Mice	CF_1	F	40	P	Chen *et al.* (1978)
	Mice	Balb/c	M	20	E	Clapp *et al.* (1984)
	Mice		M	20	E	Clapp *et al.* (1984)
DMH	Rats	Wistar	F	20	N	Cruse *et al.* (1978)
	Rats		M	3.8 g/kcal	P	Kroes *et al.* (1986)
DMH	Rats	Sprague–Dawley	F	20	N	Barbolt and Abraham (1980)
	Rats		M	20	P	
	Rats		M	20	P	Wilson *et al.* (1977)
	Rats		M	20	P	Barbolt and Abraham (1978)
	Rats		M	20	N	Bauer *et al.* (1979)
	Rats		M	20	P	Abraham *et al.* (1980)
	Rats		M	20	E	Jacobs (1983)
	Rats		M	20	P	Jacobs (1983)
	Rats	Chester–Beatty	M	28	P	Fleiszer *et al.* (1978)
	Rats	F344	M	20	P	Barnes *et al.* (1983)
	Rats	F344	M	15	E	Pence *et al.* (1986)
AOM	Rats	Sprague–Dawley				
AOM	Rats	Fischer 344	F	15	P	Watanabe *et al.* (1979)
DMH	Rats	Sprague–Dawley	M	6.5	E	Bauer *et al.* (1979)
	Rats	Wistar	M	4.5	N	Freeman *et al.* (1980)
	Rats	Wistar	M	9.0	N	Freeman *et al.* (1980)
	Rats	Sprague–Dawley	M	5.0 HM	E	Bauer *et al.* (1981)
	Rats	Sprague–Dawley	M	5.0 LM	E	Bauer *et al.* (1981)
	Rats	Sprague–Dawley	M	10	E	Jacobs and Lupton (1986)
MNU	Rats	Fischer 344	F	15	N	Watanabe *et al.* (1979)

Notes: [a]HM, high methoxylated; LM, low methoxylated.
[b]E, enhancement; N, no effect; P, protective.

was correlated with a pH lowering effect (Jacobs and Lupton, 1986). For pectin the data are contradictory, but several experiments with DMH-treated rats show tumour enhancement. Studies of the effects of miscellaneous fibres on tumour induction in rodent models suggest that the effect of specific dietary fibre is related to its physicochemical properties. In general, those fibres that are more insoluble and less fermentable, such as cellulose and wheat bran, are the most successful at inhibiting tumour development. This is in contrast to the viscous and more fermentable fibres, such as the pectins and gums, which for the most part have been associated with increased tumour incidence.

There is also known to be a direct correlation between faecal bile concentration and fibre. Cellulose and wheat bran both reduce faecal bile concentration and tumour development, whilst corn bran and oat bran increase faecal bile acid and enhance tumourigenesis. However, pectin, agar, guar gum and alfalfa are exceptions to this pattern as they enhance colorectal cancer without enhancing bile acid concentrations (Story, 1986). This is because another factor in the equation appears to be fibre fermentability. The fibres that inhibit tumourigenesis are the ones that are poorly fermented, whilst those that enhance it are highly fermentable.

As mentioned previously, intestinal cell proliferation also has a part to play. In the colon wheat bran, pectin and guar gum produce the greatest mucosal growth effects in the absence (Jacobs and White, 1983; Jacobs and Lupton, 1984) and presence (Jacobs, 1984; Jacobs and Lupton, 1986) of carcinogen treatment. Dietary fibre stimulation of cell proliferation is mediated in part through large bowel fermentation by anaerobic microflora, the production of short-chain fatty acids and the lowering of luminal pH (Cummings, 1983). All of these stimulate colonic cell proliferation (Sakata and Yajima, 1984; Lupton *et al.*, 1985). However, dietary cellulose in one very thoroughly executed study (Cameron *et al.*, 1989), suppressed the DMH-induced increase in mitotic activity in the colonic crypts of rats.

Colorectal bacteria

Much of the information on the metabolic activities of the flora of the digestive tract comes from animal studies. In studies in which rats are given either DMH or AOM the rate of tumour development is very much slower in the germ-free and antibiotic-treated rats than in conventional rats (Reddy *et al.*, 1974; Goldin and Gorbach, 1981). This can be explained in terms of the metabolism of a range of substrates with possible relevance to carcinogenesis. One mechanism is thought to be the metabolism of glucoronide-bound carcinogens with the release of active compounds (Goldin and Gorbach, 1983) and another the action of nitrate reductase on dietary nitrate to produce nitrite, an essential precursor of endogenous *N*-nitrosation (Hill, 1989 and references therein). A number of amino acids are also metabolised *in vivo* to produce compounds that are known to be carcinogens, co-carcinogens, tumour promoters, mutagens or co-mutagens. Tyrosine is metabolised in the gut to produce volatile phenols, and tryptophan is metabolised in humans to a wide range of products all of which could be produced by the gut bacterial flora. Also, we know from the previous section that bile acids are extensively metabolised in the colon to give deoxycholate and lithocholic acid, both of which have been shown to be tumour promoters in animal studies (Narisawa *et al.*, 1974; Reddy and Watanabe, 1979; Sarwal *et al.*, 1979; Cohen *et al.*, 1980).

Ethanol

Both epidemiological studies and animal experiments have identified ethanol as a co-carcinogen for various organs including the rectum (Seitz and Simanowski, 1988). Some of the epidemiological data are presented in Chapter 3.

Ethanol *per se* is not a carcinogen (Ketcham *et al.*, 1963) and in at least three studies in rats has been shown to have no effect on DMH-induced colorectal carcinogenesis irrespective of whether it was administered in the drinking water (Nelson and Samelson, 1985; Howarth and Pihl, 1985) or as a liquid diet (McGarrity *et al.*, 1987). However, when administered to certain animals in combination with a chemical carcinogen it can enhance tumours of the rectum (Seitz *et al.*, 1984; Garzon *et al.*, 1987*a*) or inhibit tumour formation (Hamilton, 1987*a*, *b*; Seitz *et al.*, 1987*a*) dependent on the dose. Ethanol was shown to affect carcinogenesis during the pre-induction and/or induction phase including carcinogen metabolism, but not during the post-induction phase (promotion). Also, since chronic administration of ethanol either as a liquid diet (Garzon *et al.*, 1987*a*) or intragastrically (Seitz *et al.*, 1987*b*) accelerates the rectal tumours induced by acetoxymethyl-methylnitrosamine (AMMN) it seems that alcohol enhances carcinogenesis, at least in part, by local mechanisms in the rectal mucosa and not by increasing the activation of pro-carcinogens. However, it is known that ethanol inhibits the hepatic microsomal activation of AOM (Sohn *et al.*, 1987) and of DMN (Peng *et al.*, 1982; Sohn *et al.*, 1987).

Inhibitors of colorectal carcinogenesis

Natural inhibitors

Selenium This trace element, shown in epidemiological studies to provide a protective effect against colorectal carcinoma (Clark, 1985), inhibits colon carcinogenesis in rats treated with DMH or MAM (Jacobs *et al.*, 1977; Soullier *et al.*, 1981). However, the effect was only seen at selenium concentrations that were slightly toxic, as assessed by decreased weight gain, and far in excess of those required for normal nutrition. The effect was also dependent on the dose of DMH, with the greatest inhibition of carcinogenesis being seen at the lower doses. The mechanism of selenium inhibition is unknown, but the fact that it is not organ specific suggests a generalised systemic mechanism. The dominant theory is that because selenium is an essential component of glutathione peroxidase it protects the cells against oxidative damage (Lane and Medina, 1983). Selenium at high concentration is also known to depress cell proliferation (Le Boeuf and Hoekstra, 1985).

Calcium Inhibition of intestinal carcinogenesis by dietary calcium has been studied in several animal models. In studies in which two different strains of rats and two different doses of AOM were used, high calcium supplementation failed to inhibit tumourigenesis, irrespective of whether the animals were maintained on high-fat or low-fat diets (Nigro and Bull, 1989). However, calcium was shown to reduce the incidence of DMH-induced tumours in rats from 86 per cent in the low calcium group to 53 per cent in the high calcium group, but only in animals consuming a 20 per cent corn oil diet (Pence and Buddingh, 1987). Therefore the role of calcium in preventing colon tumourigenesis remains uncertain.

Vitamins Ascorbate (vitamin C) has been studied as a chemopreventive agent in individuals with FPC (FAP) (Bussey *et al.*, 1982) and some vitamins appear to inhibit cancer when they are given in amounts greater than those required for the maintenance of general health or as supplements to eliminate a vitamin deficiency (Bertram *et al.*, 1987). Generally vitamins C and E are proposed as anticarcinogenic agents because of their antioxidant properties. Reddy *et al.* (1982) reported that 1 per cent ascorbate administered in the diet inhibited tumourigenesis following a single dose of DMH. It had no effect on carcinogenesis induced by multiple doses of DMH or MNU. Mice fed 0.06 per cent vitamin E showed reduced DMH-induced colon tumourigenesis (Cook and McNamara, 1980).

Vitamin A and related retinoids administered in the diet after carcinogenic treatment have been reported to reduce DMH- and MNU-induced tumourigenesis in rats (Newberne and Suphakarn, 1977; Silverman *et al.*, 1981), although reduced food consumption and body weight may have contributed to the effect. Retinoids had no effect on MNU-induced tumourigenesis in another study. A deficiency of vitamin A increased aflatoxin B induced colon carcinogenesis (Newberne and Rogers, 1973).

Plant sterols Epidemiological studies indicate that vegetarians have a lower colon cancer incidence than the general population living in the same area, which it has been suggested might be due to the sterol content of vegetables. Vegetables are rich in plant sterols (Subbish, 1971) and plant sterols are known to prevent cholesterol absorption and reduce serum cholesterol levels in both rats and humans. A 0.2 per cent β-sitosterol supplement to the diet of MNNG-treated rats inhibited both the incidence and frequency of tumours compared with the animals not receiving the supplement (Raicht *et al.*, 1980). However, although the total number of tumours was dramatically reduced from 50 per cent to 33 per cent, the number of invasive carcinomas remained the same in both the treated and the control animals. Raicht *et al.* (1980) concluded, therefore, that β-sitosterol might prevent adenoma formation, but not the transition from adenoma to carcinoma. Some support for this thesis comes from the studies of Deschner *et al.* (1982), who demonstrated that supplementation of the diet of rats with β-sitosterol slowed epithelial proliferation in both carcinogen- and non-carcinogen-treated animals. This suggests a mechanism for the reduction of both pre-neoplastic adenomas and neoplastic carcinomas.

Others Diallyl sulphide (DAS), a major component of garlic oil, was shown to inhibit intestinal carcinogenesis when given to mice prior to the administration of DMH (Wargovich, 1987). Naturally occurring protease inhibitors, such as the Bowman–Birk inhibitor, have been shown to reduce the tumour incidence in mice treated with DMH (Weed *et al.*, 1985). Sodium cyanate, which is structurally related to several naturally occurring inhibitors in cruciferous vegetables, has also been shown to inhibit DMH-induced tumours when added to the diet after carcinogen treatment (Wattenberg, 1984).

Synthetic inhibitors

Phenols These compounds are antioxidants which occur naturally in plants and have been reported to possess carcinogenic inhibitory properties. Butylated hydroxyanisole (BHA) and butylated hydroxytoluene (BHT) are two synthetic phenolic antioxidants which are widely used as food additives. Both BHA and BHT are potent inhibitors of polycyclic aromatic hydrocarbon-induced tumourigenesis in animals. However, the results for the colon are inconclusive (Wattenberg, 1985). BHT administered in the diet inhibited AOM-induced intestinal tumours in rats (Weisburger *et al.*, 1977). BHT failed to inhibit DMH-induced colon tumours in a different strain of rat (Barbolt and Abraham, 1977).

Administration of BHA to mice concurrently with the carcinogen was reported to reduce tumour incidence. Thus, phenolic antioxidants may inhibit colon carcinogenesis, but the mechanism is unresolved (Bull *et al.*, 1981).

Disulfiram This is a potent inhibitor of the conversion of DMH to AOM (Fiala *et al.*, 1977), but also inhibits AOM-induced tumourigenesis in rats (Nigro and Campbell, 1978) suggesting that it acts too at another point in the pathway. It is difficult to see what extrapolations can be made from these studies to colon carcinogenesis in humans.

Difluoromethylornithine Ornithine decarboxylase (ODC) is the rate-limiting enzyme in polyamine biosynthesis. Polyamine levels and polyamine pathway enzyme activities are high in proliferating cells and in cells undergoing neoplastic change (Luk *et al.*, 1986). Increased ODC activity is also seen in mouse skin following treatment with the tumour promoter 12-*O*-tetradecanoylphorbol-13-acetate (TPA) (O'Brien *et al.*, 1975; Yuspa *et al.*, 1976) and in the colonic mucosa following the administration of chronic dietary ethanol (Hamilton and Luk, 1987). Difluoromethylornithine (DFMO) is an irreversible inhibitor of ODC activity. DFMO (1 per cent) administered in the drinking water of DMH-treated mice reduced both the colon polyamine levels and the incidence of colon tumours (Kingsnorth *et al.*, 1983). DFMO (0.1–1.0 per cent) reduced colon tumour incidence in AOM-treated rats (Rozhin *et al.*, 1984). The data although limited suggest that DFMO is a useful inhibitor of tumourigenesis, particularly as it is non-toxic.

Prostaglandin inhibitors It has been suggested that tumour initiation, promotion and metastasis may require prostaglandin biosynthesis (Honn *et al.*, 1981). Indomethacin, a non-steroidal anti-inflammatory drug, is known to reduce the formation of prostaglandins. Intrarectal administration of indomethacin following chemical induction of tumours showed indomethacin to inhibit their growth (Kudo *et al.*, 1980). Narisawa *et al.* (1978) had shown previously that early intraperitoneal administration of indomethacin inhibited colon tumour growth whilst late administration reduced the size of the tumours that had already developed. The drug was also found to be effective when given orally in the drinking water (Narisawa *et al.*, 1981; Pollard and Luckert, 1983), although tumours reappeared rapidly once the treatment was stopped. Similar data were obtained for the less toxic prostaglandin inhibitor piroxicam (Pollard *et al.*, 1983). However, one study (Danzi *et al.*, 1984) has shown indomethacin to increase animal mortality and increase metastasis.

Evaluation of new chemotherapeutic agents

To date chemotherapeutic research has largely involved clinical trials of empirical cytotoxic drug regimes of necessity on patients with advanced disease. Of the more than 40 chemotherapeutic agents evaluated in the treatment of colorectal cancer, only three classes have been shown to exert limited activity: the fluoropyrimidines, which are pyrimidine antagonists; the nitrosoureas, which inhibit protein, DNA and RNA synthesis; and mitomycin C, which is a crosslinking agent.

It is obvious, therefore, that studies of the effects of chemotherapy on colorectal carcinoma would be greatly facilitated by the availability of suitable animal models. Originally two experimental approaches to the problem of colorectal chemotherapy were used. The first utilised human colon tumour xenografts in immunodeficient mice (Cobb and Mitchley, 1974; Lamberton and Steele, 1975; Tibbetts *et al.*, 1977) and the second the serial transplantation of colon tumours induced in mice by DMH (Ball and Double, 1975; Griswald and Corbett, 1975; Corbett *et al.*, 1977). In neither of these systems were the tumours autochthonous to the host or even sited in the gastrointestinal tract. Now the studies are performed on autochthonous rodent colon cancer models (Sych *et al.*, 1978). Studies of the effect of the combination chemotherapy of 5-fluorouracil (5-FU) and 1,3-bis(2-chloroethyl)-1-nitrosourea (BCNU) on DMH-induced tumours in rats showed chemotherapy to prolong significantly the survival of the rats with the least advanced disease, but to have no effect on locally advanced metastatic disease (Danzi *et al.*, 1983).

Such studies are considered to mimic the human situation better than transplantable tumours (Zeller and Berger, 1984). Titanium complexes showed a dose-dependent inhibition of tumour growth (Bischoff, Thesis 1986, University of Heidelberg). Ruthenium derivatives strongly inhibited tumour growth (Garzon *et al.*, 1987*a*). Flavoacetic acid and 5′-deoxy-5-fluorouridine showed strong antitumour effects, which were synergistic in combination at non-toxic doses (Garzon *et al.*, 1989). Similar antitumour activity was observed for 4-amino-*N*(2′-aminophenyl)benzamide.

Animal models and their relevance to human colorectal cancer

Very fortuitously the animal models for colorectal carcinogenesis seem to resemble very closely the human situation in their histopathology (Shamsuddin, 1983; Teague, 1983; Nakamura and Kino, 1985). Dysplastic crypts can be seen in sections of colons from animals subjected to repeated carcinogen treatment (Deschner *et al.*, 1979; Chang, 1984) and in humans predisposed to colon carcinoma, i.e. individuals with FPC (FAP) or long-standing ulcerative colitis (Riddell, 1984). Animal models have therefore provided an insight into the mechanisms by which the agents and factors identified by the epidemiologists in Chapter 3 modulate the risk of the disease, mainly by facilitating a level of experimentation that would be unacceptable in humans. Moreover, the experimental systems are becoming more sophisticated all the time. Recently, Povey, O'Neill and co-workers have developed a non-invasive, microcapsule system to scavenge electrophilic species and study the effects of previously identified dietary modulators of carcinogenesis on both administered and endogenous DNA damaging agents (Povey *et al.*, 1987; O'Neill *et al.*, 1987, 1988). The same studies evaluated the use of human diets in rodents. More recently still, a system for identifying foci of aberrant crypts in mice and rats in response to food-related carcinogens has been reported (Tudek *et al.*, 1989) which looks especially promising for the identification of the components of the human diet that might be responsible for the origin of colorectal cancer.

This is important, because our understanding of the components of the initiation and promotion processes involved in human colorectal cancer still has very significant gaps (Table 4.4; Weisburger *et al.*, 1989). This is particularly true with regard to the identification of the initiating carcinogens. Bruce (1987) discovered relatively powerful direct-acting mutagens in the stools of some individuals which were identified as faecapentaenes. Unfortunately, pure faecapentaenes in contact with the intestinal epithelium failed to induce micronuclei (Bruce, 1987), although in *in vitro* cell systems they were shown to be DNA damaging (Curren *et al.*, 1987; Hinzman *et al.*, 1987). Also, as mentioned previously (Chapter 3), Sugimura (1985) has demonstrated that powerful mutagens are formed during the cooking processes for meat and fish. However, the amounts of these carcinogens found in fried foods are small and may not have a significant role to play in the overall generation of colorectal cancer. The indications are that animal models such as those described above and those in which animals are subjected to endoscopic examination at various stages following carcinogen treatment (Narisawa *et al.*, 1975) will provide the key to the identification of the carcinogenic threat to humans.

How useful animal models will be for studies of chemotherapeutic agents, immunological responses and immunotherapy (Sjorgen and Steele, 1975) is less clear. Certainly with regard to the study of the effects of chemotherapeutic agents it is clear that the differences in drug metabolism between animals and humans are really quite marked. Nowhere is

Table 4.4. *Mechanism postulated for aetiological factors bearing on segments of large bowel cancer*

Disease	Carcinogen	Promoting elements	Protective elements	Suggested mechanisms
Hereditary adenomatosis Familial polyposis Gardner's syndrome	Cellular genome	?	Victamin C?	Genetically mediated programme towards neoplasia
Ulcerative colitis	?	Refined carbohydrates	Cereal fibre, calcium salts, low-fat diets Ceareal	Higher cell turnover rates favour carcinogenesis
Crohn's disease	?	Refined carbohydrates, smoking	Cereal fibre, calcium salts, low-fat diets	
High-risk non-polyposis	Fried food?	Dietary fat (bile and fatty acids)	Cereal fibre, calcium salts, yellow-green vegetables, low-fat diets	Higher cell turnover; other mechanisms may be similar to those for distal colon cancer
Proximal colon neoplasms?	?	Dietary fat (bile and fatty acids)? Oestrogen? Obesity? Cholecystectomy?	Cereal fibre, calcium salts, yellow-green vegetables?	?
Distal colon neoplasms	Fried food	Dietary fat (bile and fatty acids)	Cereal fibre, calcium salts, yellow-green vegetables, olive oil, fish oils	Initation by carcinogens produced during cooking; also postulated are mutagens stemming from specific bacterial cell membranes. Enhancement (promotion) by bile and fatty acids related to total fat intake (except olive and fish oils). Protection by stool bulk (cereal fibre), calcium binding of bile or fatty acids, or unknown mechanisms through yellow-green vegetables, control of cell proliferation by calcium or suitable lower pH
Rectal neoplasms?	?	Dietary fat? Alcohol?	Cereal fibre? Calcium salts?	Some data show parallel, but not identical, factors as for distal colon cancer. However, there are also sharply distinct elements. Basically unknown mechanisms, although effects on cell duplication rates are relevant

this better demonstrated than in the studies of the therapeutic efficacy of the cytotoxic drug *N*-(phosphonacetyl)L-aspartate (PALA). Although very effective against tumours at various sites in rodents (Johnson *et al.*, 1976, 1978) it has been shown to be essentially ineffective in clinical trials (Ervin *et al.*, 1980; Creagan, 1981*a*, *b*; Kleeberg *et al.*, 1982). This may in part be explained by studies using *in vitro* human fibroblast cultures, where the efficiency of the salvage pathways in the tumour cell lines confers increased drug resistance (Kinsella and Haran, 1991).

With regard to the immunology of the disease, there is no association between immunodeficiency and colorectal cancer (Filipovich *et al.*, 1980) and studies in which monoclonal antibodies are used for tumour detection are very few (Sjorgen and Steele, 1975; Lynch and Salomon, 1979; McCabe *et al.*, 1988).

References

Abraham, R., Barbolt, T. A. and Rodgers, J. B. (1980) Inhibition by bran of the colonic co-carcinogenicity of bile salts in rats given dimethylhydrazine. *Exp. Mol. Pathol.*, **33**, 133–45.

Autrup, H. and Williams, G. M. (1983) Carcinogenesis studies in human gastrointestinal epithelium. In: *Experimental Colon Carcinogenesis*, ed. H. Autrup, and G. M. Williams, pp. 95–106. CRC Press, Boca Raton.

Ball, C. R. and Double, J. A. (1975) Transplantable colon tumours as chemotherapy screening models. *Cancer*, **36**, 2437–40.

Bansal, B. R., Rhoads, J. E. and Bansal, S. C. (1978) Effects of diet on colon carcinogenesis and the immune system in rats treated with 1,2-dimethylhydrazine. *Cancer Res.*, **38**, 3293–303.

Barbolt, T. A. and Abraham, R. (1977) Lack of effect of butylated hydroxytoluene on dimethylhydrazine-induced colon carcinogenesis in rats. *Experientia*, **35**, 257–8.

Barbolt, T. A. and Abraham, R. (1978) The effect of bran on dimethylhydrazine-induced colon carcinogenesis in the rat. *Proc. R. Soc. Med.*, **157**, 656–9.

Barbolt, T. A. and Abraham, R. (1980) Dose–response, sex difference and the effect of bran in dimethylhydrazine-induced intestinal tumourigenesis in rats. *Toxicol. Appl. Pharmacol.*, **55**, 417–22.

Barnes, D. S., Clapp, N. K., Scott, S. A., *et al.* (1983) Effects of wheat, rice, corn and soybean bran on 1,2-dimethylhydrazine-induced large bowel tumourigenesis in F344 rats. *Nutr. Cancer*, **5**, 1–9.

Barton, T., Cruse, J. P. and Lewin, M. R. (1987) Changes in serum lipids related to the presence of experimental colon cancer. *Br. J. Cancer*, **56**, 451–4.

Bauer, H. G., Asp, N.-G., Dahlquist, A. and Fredlund, P. E. (1979) Effect of dietary fiber on the induction of colorectal tumours and fecal β-glucuronidase activity in the rat. *Cancer Res.*, **39**, 3725–56.

Bauer, H. G., Asp, N.-G., Dahlquist, A., *et al.* (1981) Effects of two kinds of pectin and guar gum on 1,2-dimethylhydrazine initiation of colon tumours and on fecal β-glucuronidase activity in the rat. *Cancer Res.*, **41**, 2518–23.

Bertram, J. S., Kolonel, L. N. and Meyskens, F. L. (1987) Rationale and strategies for chemoprevention of cancer in humans. *Cancer Res.*, **47**, 3012–31.

Broitman, S. A. (1986) Cholesterol, conundrums: the relationship between dietary and serum cholesterol in colon cancer. In: *Dietary Fat and Cancer*, ed. I. P. Clement *et al.*, pp. 435–59. A. R. Liss, New York.

Broitman, S. A., Vitale, J. J., Vavrousek-Jakuba, E. and Gottlieb, L. S. (1977) Polyunsaturated fat, cholesterol and large bowel tumourigenesis. *Cancer*, **40**, 2455–63.

Bruce, W. R. (1986) What chemicals are responsible for colon cancer? *J. Cell Physiol.*, **4**, 47–9.

Bruce, W. R. (1987) Recent hypotheses for the origin of colon cancer. *Cancer Res.*, **47**, 4237–42.

Bull, A. W., Burd, A. D. and Nigro, N. D. (1979) Promotion of azoxymethane-induced intestinal cancer by high fat diets in rats. *Cancer Res.*, **39**, 4956–9.

Bull, A. W., Burd, A. D. and Nigro, N. D. (1981) Effects of inhibitors of tumourigenesis on the formation of O^6-methylguanine in the colon of 1,2-dimethylhydrazine-treated rats. *Cancer Res.*, **41**, 4938–41.

Bussey, H. J., De Cosse, J. and Deschner, E. F., *et al.* (1982) A randomised trial of ascorbic acid in polyposis coli. *Cancer*, **50**, 1434–9.

Cameron, I. L., Ord, V. A., Hunter, K. E., *et al.* (1989) Suppression of carcinogen (1,2-dimethylhydrazine dichloride)-induced increase in mitotic activity in the colonic crypts of rats by addition of dietary cellulose. *Cancer Res.*, **49**, 991–5.

Chang, W. W. L. (1984) Histogenesis of colon cancer in experimental animals. *Scand. J. Gastroenterol.*, **19**, 27–43.

Chen, W.-F., Patchefsky, A. S. and Goldsmith, H. S. (1978) Colonic protection from dimethylhydrazine by a high fiber diet. *Surg. Gynecol. Obstet.*, **147**, 503–6.

Clapp, N. K., Henke, M. A., London, J. F. and Shock, T. L. (1984) Enhancement of 1,2-dimethylhydrazine-induced large bowel tumourigenesis in Balb/C mice by corn, soybean and wheat brans. *Nutr. Cancer*, **6**, 77–85.

Clark, L. C. (1985) The epidemiology of selenium and cancer. *Fed. Proc.*, **44**, 2584–9.

Cobb, L. M. and Mitchley, B. C. V. (1974) Development of a method for assessing the antitumour activity of the chemotherapeutic agents using human xenografts. *Cancer Chemother. Rep.*, **58**, 645–51.

Cohen, B. I., Raicht, R. F., Deschner, E. E., *et al.* (1980) Effect of cholic acid feeding on *N*-methyl-*N*-nitrosourea induced colon tumours and cell kinetics in rats. *J. Natl. Cancer Inst.*, **64**, 573–8.

Committee on Diet, Nutrition and Cancer (1982) National Academy Press Washington, DC, pp. 515–33.

Cook, M. G. and McNamara, P. (1980) Effect of dietary vitamin E on dimethylhydrazine induced colonic tumours in mice. *Cancer Res.*, **40**, 1329–31.

Cooper, H. K., Buecheler, J. and Kleihues, P. (1978) DNA alkylation in mice with genetically different susceptibility. *Cancer Res.*, **38**, 3063–5.

Corbett, T. H., Griswold, D. P., Roberts, B. J., *et al.* (1977) Evaluation of single agents and combinations of agents. *Cancer*, **40**, 2660–80.

Core, S. K. and Watne, A. L. (1974) Faecal steroids and colon cancer. *Fed. Proc.*, **33**, 260.

Creagan, E. T., Ahmann, D. L., Ingle, J. N., *et al.* (1981*a*) Phase II evaluation of

PALA and AMSA for patients with disseminated malignant melanoma. *Cancer Treat. Rep.*, **65**, 169.

Creagan, E. T., Eagan, R. T., Fleming, T. R., *et al.* (1981*b*) Phase II evaluation of PALA in patients with metastatic lung cancer. *Cancer Treat. Rep.*, **65**, 356–7.

Cruse, J. P. (1989) Cholesterol, neutral sterols and colorectal cancer. In: *Colorectal Cancer*, ed. H. K. Seitz, U. A. Simanowski and N. A. Wright, pp. 112–24. Springer, Berlin.

Cruse, J. P., Lewin, M. R. and Clark, C. G. (1978*a*) Failure of bran to protect against experimental colon cancer in rats. *Lancet*, **2**, 1278–80.

Cruse, J. P., Lewin, M. R., Ferulano, G. P. and Clark, G. G. (1978*b*) Cocarcinogenic effects of dietary cholesterol in experimental colon cancer. *Nature*, **276**, 822–5.

Cummings, J. H. (1983) Fermentation in the human large intestine: evidence and implications for health. *Lancet*, **1**, 1206–11.

Curren, R. D., Putman, D. L., Yang, L. L., *et al.* (1987) Genotoxicity of faecapentane-12 in bacterial and mammalian cell assay systems. *Carcinogenesis*, **8**, 349–52.

Danzi, M., Lewin, M. R., Cruse, J. P. and Clark C. G. (1983) Combination chemotherapy with 5-fluorouracil (5FU) and 1,3-bis(2-chloro-ethyl)-1-nitrosourea (BCNU) prolongs survival of rats with dimethylhydrazine induced colon cancer. *Gut*, **24**, 1041–7.

Danzi, M., Ferulano, G. P., Abate, S. and Califano, G. (1984) Enhancement of colonic cancer by indomethacin treatment in dimethylhydrazine pretreated rats. *Carcinogenesis*, **5**, 287–9.

Deschner, E. E. (1985) Cell kinetic approaches to defining premalignant conditions. In: *Carcinoma of the Large Bowel and its Precursors*, ed. J. R. F. Ingall and J. Mastromarino, pp. 187–202. A. R. Liss, New York.

Deschner, E. E. and Masken, A. P. (1983) Significance of the labelling distribution as kinetic parameters in colorectal mucosa of cancer patients and DMH-treated animals. *Cancer*, **50**, 1136–41.

Deschner, E. E., Long, F. C. and Maskens, A. P. (1979) Relationship between dose, time and tumour yield in mouse dimethylhydrazine-induced colon tumourigenesis. *Cancer Lett.*, **8**, 23–8.

Deschner, E. E., Cohen, B. I. and Raicht, R. F. (1982) The kinetics of the protective effect of β-sitosterol against MNU-induced colonic neoplasia. *J. Cancer Res. Clin. Oncol.*, **103**, 49–54.

Druckrey, H., Preussman, S. and Ivanbovic, D., *et al.* (1967) Organotropic carcinogenic effects of 65 *N*-nitroso compounds on BD rats. *Z. Krebsforsch.*, **69**, 103–201.

El Khatib, S. M. and Cora, E. M. (1981) Role of high fat diet in tumourigenesis in C57 B2/1 mice. *J. Natl. Canc. Inst.*, **66**, 297–301.

Ervin, T. J., Blum, R. H., Meshad, M. W., *et al.* (1980) Phase I trial of *N*-(phosphonacetyl)-L-aspartic acid (PALA). *Cancer Treat. Rep.*, **64**, 1067–71.

Farber, E. (1984) Cellular biochemistry of the stepwise development of cancer with chemicals. *Cancer Res.*, **44**, 5463–74.

Fiala, E. S., Bobotas, G. and Kulakis, C., *et al.* (1977) Effects of disulfram and related compounds on the metabolism in vivo of the colon carcinogen 1,2-dimethylhydrazine. *Biochem. Pharmacol.*, **26**, 1763–8.

Filipovich, A. H., Spector, B. D. and Kersey, J. (1980) Immunodeficiency in humans as a risk factor in the development of malignancy. *Prev. Med.*, **9**, 252–9.

Fleiszer, D., Murray, D., McFarlane, J. and Brown, R. A. (1978) Protective effect of dietary fibre against chemically-induced bowel tumours in rats. *Lancet*, **2**, 552–3.

Freeman, H. J., Spiller, G. A. and Kim, Y. S. (1980) A double-blind study on the effects of different purified cellulose and pectin fiber diets on 1,2-dimethylhydrazine-induced rat colonic neoplasia. *Cancer Res.*, **38**, 2912–17.

Garzon, F. T., Berger, M. R., Keppler, B. K. and Schmahl, D. (1987*a*) Comparative anti-tumour activity of ruthenium derivatives with 5′deoxy-5-fluorouridine in chemically induced colorectal tumours in SD rats. *Cancer Chemother. Pharmacol.*, **19**, 347–9.

Garzon, F. T., Simanowski, U. A. and Berger, M. R., *et al.* (1987*b*) Acetoxymethyl-methylnitrosamine (AMMN)-induced colorectal carcinogenesis is stimulated by chronic alcohol consumption. *Alcohol*, **1**, 501–2.

Garzon, F. T., Berger, M. R. and Schmahl, D. (1989) Experimental models to study new chemotherapeutic agents in colorectal cancer. In: *Colorectal Cancer*, ed. H. K. Seitz, U. A. Simanowksi and N. A. Wright, pp. 349–58. Springer, Berlin.

Glickman, L. T., Suissa, S. and Fleizer, D. M. (1987) Proliferative characteristics of colonic crypt cells in C57BL/6J and A/J mice as predictors of subsequent tumour formation. *Cancer Res.*, **47**, 4766–70.

Goldin, B. and Gorbach, S. L. (1981) Effects of antibiotics on incidence of rat intestinal tumours induced by 1,2-dimethylhydrazine. *J. Natl. Cancer Inst.*, **67**, 877–80.

Goldin, B. and Gorbach, S. L. (1983) Activation of carcinogens by bacterial and microsomal enzyme systems. *Gastroenterology*, **85**, 200–1.

Griswald, D. P. and Corbett, T. H. (1975) A colon tumour model for anticancer agent evaluation. *Cancer*, **36**, 2441–4.

Hamilton, S. R. and Luk, G. D. (1987) Induction of colonic mucosal ornithine decarboxylase activity by chronic dietary ethanol consumption in the rat. *Gastroenterology*, **92**, 1423.

Hamilton, S. R., Stephens, R. B., Natuzzi, E., *et al.* (1982) Morphologic analogy of intestinal tract carcinogenesis in adenomatous polyposis and azoxymethane-treated rat model. *Lab. Invest.*, **46**, 33A–34A.

Hamilton, S. R., Hyland, J., McAvinchey, D., *et al.* (1987*a*) Effects of chronic dietary beer and ethanol consumption on experimental colonic carcinogenesis induced by azoxymethane in rats. *Cancer Res.*, **47**, 1551–9.

Hamilton, S. R., Sohn, O. S. and Fiala, E. S. (1987*b*) Effects of timing and quantity of chronic dietary ethanol consumption on azoxymethane-induced colon carcinogenesis and azoxymethane metabolism in Fischer 344 rats. *Cancer Res.*, **47**, 4305–11.

Hawks, A. and Magee, D. M. (1974) The alkylation of nucleic acids in the rat and mouse in vivo by the carcinogen 1,2-dimethylhydrazine. *Br. J. Cancer*, **30**, 440–7.

Heitman, D. W., Grubbs, B. G., Heitman, T. O. and Cameron, I. L. (1983) Effects of 1,2-dimethylhydrazine treatment and feeding regimen on rat colonic epithelial cell proliferation. *Cancer Res.*, **43**, 1153–62.

Hill, M. J. (1989) Colorectal bacteria in colorectal carcinogenesis. In: *Colorectal Cancer*, ed. H. K. Seitz, U. A. Simanowski and N. A. Wright, pp. 160–76. Springer, Berlin.

Hill, M. J., Morson, B. C. and Thompson, M. H. (1983) The role of faecal bile acids (FBA) in large bowel carcinogenesis. *Br. J. Cancer*, **48**, 143.

Hinzman, M. J., Novotny, C., Ullah, A. and Shamsuddin, A. M. (1987) Faecal mutagen faecapentane-12 damages mammalian colon epithelial DNA. *Carcinogenesis*, **8**, 1475–9.

Hiramatsu, Y., Takada, H., Yamamura, M., Hioki, K., Saito, K. and Yamamoto, M. (1983) Effect of dietary cholesterol on azoxymethane-induced colon carcinogenesis in rats. *Carcinogenesis*, **4**, 553–8.

Hofmann, A. F. (1977) The enterohepatic circulation of bile acids in man. *Clin. Gastoenterol.*, **6**, 3–24.

Honn, K. V., Brockman, R. S. and Marnett, L. J. (1981) Prostaglandins and cancer: a review of tumour initiation through metastases. *Prostaglandins*, **21**, 833–64.

Howarth, A. E. and Pihl, E. (1985) High fat diet promotes and causes distal shift of experimental colonic cancer: beer and alcohol do not. *Nutr. Cancer*, **6**, 229–35.

Isaksson, A., Lundquist, I., Akesson, B. and Ihse, I. (1984) Effect of pectin and wheat bran on intraluminal pancreatic enzyme activities and on fat absorption as examined by triolein breath test in patients with pancreatic insufficiency. *Scand. J. Gastroenterol.*, **19**, 457–73.

Jacobs, L. R. (1983) Enhancement of rat colon carcinogenesis by wheat bran consumption during the stage of 1,2-dimethylhydrazine administration. *Cancer Res.*, **43**, 4057–61.

Jacobs, L. R. (1984) Stimulation of rat colonic crypt cell proliferative activity by wheat bran consumption during the stage of 1,2-dimethylhydrazine administration. *Cancer Res.*, **44**, 2458–63.

Jacobs, L. R. and Lupton, J. R. (1984) Effect of dietary fibres on rat large bowel mucosal growth and cell proliferation. *Am. J. Physiol.*, **246**, 378–85.

Jacobs, L. R. and Lupton, J. R. (1986) Relationship between colon luminal pH, cell proliferation and colon carcinogenesis in 1,2-dimethylhydrazine treated rats fed high fibre diets. *Cancer Res.*, **46**, 1727–34.

Jacobs, L. R. and White, F. A. (1983) Modulation of mucosal cell proliferation in the intestine of rats fed a wheat bran diet. *Am. J. Clin. Nutr.*, **37**, 945–53.

Jacobs, M. M., Jansson, B. and Griffin, A. C. (1977) Inhibitory effects of selenium on 1,2-dimethylhydrazine and methylazoxymethanol acetate induction of colon tumours. *Cancer Lett.*, **2**, 133–8.

Jain, M., Cook, G. M., David, F. G., *et al.* (1980) A case control study of diet and colorectal cancer. *Int. J. Cancer*, **26**, 757–68.

Johnson, R. K., Inouye, T., Goldin, A. and Stark, G. R. (1976) Antitumour activity of *N*-phosphonacetyl-L-aspartic acid, a transition state inhibitor of aspartate transcarbamylase. *Cancer Res.*, **36**, 2720–5.

Johnson, R. K., Swyryd, E. A. and Stark, G. R. (1978) Effects of *N*-phosphonacetyl-L-aspartate on murine tumours and normal tissues in vitro and in vivo and the relationship of sensitivity to rate of proliferation and level of aspartate transcarbamylase. *Cancer Res.*, **38**, 371–8.

Kaur, A. P., Bhat, C. M. and Grewal, R. B. (1985) Effect of cellulose incorporation in a low fibre diet of faecal excretion and digestibility of nutrients in adolescent girls. *Nutr. Rep. Int.*, **32**, 383–90.

Ketcham, A. S., Wexler, H. and Mantel, N. (1963) Effects of alcohol in mouse neoplasia. *Cancer Res.*, **23**, 667–70.

Kingsnorth, A. N., King, W. W. K. and Diekma, K. A., *et al.* (1983) Inhibition of ornithine decarboxylase with 2-difluoromethylornithine: reduced incidence of dimethylhydrazine induced colon tumours in mice. *Cancer Res.*, **43**, 2545–9.

Kleeberg, U. R., Mulder, J. H., Rumke, P., *et al.* (1982) *N*-(phosphonacetyl)-L-aspartate in advanced malignant melanoma: a phase II trial of the EORTC Malignant Melanoma Co-operative Group. *Eur. J. Clin. Oncol.*, **18**, 723–6.

Klurfeld, D. M., Aglow, E., Tepper, S. and Kritchevsky, D. (1983) Modification of dimethylhydrazine induced carcinogenesis in rats by dietary cholesterol. *Nutr. Cancer*, **5**, 16–25.

Kroes, R., Beems, R. B., Bosland, M. C., *et al.* (1986) Nutritional factors in lung, colon and prostate carcinogenesis in animal models. *Fed. Proc. Fed. Am. Soc. Exp. Biol.*, **45**, 136–41.

Kudo, T., Narisawa, T. and Abo, S. (1980) Antitumour activity of indomethacin on methylazoxymethanol-induced large bowel tumours in rats. *Gann*, **71**, 260–4.

Lamberton, L. F. and Steele, G. G. (1975) Growth kinetics of human large bowel cancer growing in immune deprived mice and some chemotherapeutic observations. *Cancer*, **36**, 2431–6.

LaMont, J. T. and O'Gorman, T. A. (1978) Experimental colon cancer. *Gastroenterology*, **75**, 1157–69.

Lane, H. W. and Medina, D. (1983) Selenium concentration and glutathione peroxidase activity in normal and neoplastic development of the mouse mammary gland. *Cancer Res.*, **43**, 1558–61.

Le Boeuf, R. A. and Hoekstra, W. G. (1985) Changes in cellular glutathione levels: possible relation to selenium mediated anticarcinogenesis. *Fed. Proc.*, **44**, 2563–7.

Lilienfeld, A. M. (1981) The human fog: cancer and cholesterol. *Am. J. Epidemiol.*, **114**, 1–4.

Lipkin, M. (1983) Cell proliferation in colon carcinogenesis. In: *Experimental Colon Carcinogenesis*, ed. A. Autrup and G. M. Williams, pp. 139–54. CRC Press, Boca Raton.

Liu, K., Moss, D. and Persky, V., *et al.* (1979) Dietary cholesterol, fat and fibre and colon cancer mortality. *Lancet*, **2**, 782–5.

Locniskar, M., Nauss, K. M. and Newberne, P. M. (1983) The effect of altering the quality and quantity of dietary fat on dimethylhydrazine (DMH)-induced colon carcinogenesis in rats. *Fed. Proc.*, **42**, 801.

Luk, G. D., Hamilton, S. R. and Yang, P., *et al.* (1986) Kinetic changes in mucosal ornithine decarboxylase activity during azoxymethane-induced colonic carcinogenesis in the rat. *Cancer Res.*, **46**, 4449–52.

Lupton, J. R., Coder, D. M. and Jacobs, L. R. (1985) Influence of luminal pH on rat large bowel epithelial cell cycle. *Am. J. Physiol.*, **249**, 382–8.

Lynch, N. R. and Salomon, J.-C. (1979) Tumour growth inhibition and potentiation of immunotherapy by indomethacin in mice. *J. Natl. Cancer Inst.*, **62**, 117–21.

McCabe, R. P., Peters, L. C., Haspel, M. V., *et al.* (1988) Preclinical studies on the pharmacokinetic properties of human monoclonal antibodies to colorectal cancer and their use in the detection of tumours. *Cancer Res.*, **48**, 4348–53.

McGarrity, T. J., Via, E. A. and Colony, P. C. (1986) Changes in tissue sialic acid content and staining in dimethylhydrazine (DMH)-induced colorectal cancer: effects of ethanol. *Gastroenterology*, **90**, 1543.

McMichael, A. J., Jenson, O. M., Parkin, D. M. and Zaridze, D. G. (1984) Dietary and endogenous cholesterol and human cancer. *Epidemiol. Rev.*, **6**, 192–216.

Madara, J. L., Harte, P., Deasy, J., *et al.* (1983) Evidence for the adenoma–carcinoma sequence in dimethylhydrazine-induced neoplasms of rat intestinal epithelium. *Am. J. Pathol.*, **110**, 230–5.

Maskens, A. P. (1980) Confirmation of the two-step nature of carcinogenesis in the rat colon adenocarcinoma model. *Cancer*, **47**, 81–9.

Maskens, A. P. and Dujardin-Loits, R. (1981) Experimental adenomas and carcinomas of the large intestine behave as distinct entities: most carcinomas arise de novo in flat mucosa. *Cancer*, **47**, 81–9.

Mastromarino, A. J., Reddy, B. S. and Wynder, E. L. (1978) Faecal profiles of anaerobic microflora of large bowel cancer patients and patients with non-hereditary large bowel polyps. *Cancer Res.*, **38**, 4459–62.

Moskovitz, M., White, C., Barnett, R. N., *et al.* (1979) Diet, faecal bile acids and neutral sterols in carcinoma of the colon. *Dig. Dis. Sci.*, **24**, 746–51.

Mudd, D. G., McKelvey, S. T. D., Norwood, W., *et al.* (1980) Faecal bile acid concentrations of patients with carcinoma or increased risk of carcinoma of the large bowel. *Gut*, **21**, 587–90.

Nakamura, S. and Kuio, I. (1985) Morphogenesis of experimental colonic neoplasms induced by dimethylhydrazine. In: *Animal Models for Intestinal Disease*, ed. C. J. Pfeiffer, pp. 99–122. CRC Press, Boca Raton.

Narisawa, T. and Weisburger, J. M. (1975) Colon cancer induction in mice by intrarectal instillation of *N*-methylnitrosourea. *Proc. Soc. Exp. Biol. Med.*, **148**, 166–72.

Narisawa, T., Magadia, N. E., Weisburger, J. H. and Wynder, E. L. (1974) Promoting effect of bile acid on colon carcinogenesis after intrarectal instillation of MNNG in rat. *J. Natl. Cancer Inst.*, **53**, 1093–7.

Narisawa, T., Kono, K., Yamaguchi, T. and Takahashi, T. (1978) Cancer chemotherapy using autochthonous large bowel cancer in rats. *Gann.*, **69**, 431–5.

Narisawa, T., Sata, M., Tani, M., Kudo, T., Takahashi, T. and Goto, A. (1981) Inhibition of development of methylnitrosourea-induced rat colon tumours by indomethacin treatment. *Cancer Res.*, **41**, 1954–7.

Nauss, K. M., Locniskar, M. and Newberne, P. M. (1983) Effect of alterations in the quality and quantity of dietary fat on 1,2-dimethylhydrazine induced colon tumourigenesis in rats. *Cancer Res.*, **43**, 4083–90.

Nauss, K. M., Locniskar, M., Paulina, T. and Newberne, P. M. (1984*a*) Morphology and distribution of 1,2-dimethylhydrazine dichloride-induced colon tumours and their relationship to gut associated lymphoid tissue in the rat. *J. Natl. Cancer Inst.*, **73**, 915–34.

Nauss, N. M., Locniskar, M., Sondergaard, D. and Newberne, P. M. (1984*b*) Lack of effect of dietary fat on *N*-nitrosomethylurea (NMU)-induced colon tumourigenesis in rats. *Carcinogenesis*, **5**, 255–60.

Nauss, K. M., Breche, D. and Newberne, P. M. (1987) Effect of beef fat on DMH-induced colon tumourigenesis: influence of rat strain and nutrient composition. *J. Nutr.*, **117**, 739–47.

Nelson, R. L. and Samelson, S. L. (1985) Neither dietary ethanol nor beer augments experimental colon carcinogenesis in rats. *Dis. Colon Rectum*, **28**, 460–2.

Newberne, P. M. and Nauss, K. M. (1986) Dietary fat and colon cancer: variable results in animal models. In: *Dietary Fat and Cancer*, ed. D. F. Birt, A. E. Rogers and C. Mettlin, pp. 311–30. A. R. Liss, New York.

Newberne, P. M. and Rogers, A. E. (1973) Rat colon carcinomas associated with aflatoxin and marginal vitamin A. *J. Natl. Cancer Inst.*, **50**, 439–48.

Newberne, P. M. and Sahaphong, S. (1989) Dietary fat and colorectal cancer: experimental evidence for tumour promotion. In: *Colorectal Cancer*, ed. H. K. Seitz, U. A. Simanowski and N. A. Wright, pp. 89–111. Springer, Berlin.

Newberne, P. M. and Suphakarn, V. (1977) Preventive role of vitamin A in colon carcinogenesis in rats. *Cancer*, **40**, 2553–6.

Nigro, N. D. and Bull, A. W. (1989) Inhibitors of colorectal carcinogenesis: experimental and therapeutic agents. In: *Colorectal Cancer*, ed. H. K. Seitz, U. A. Simonowski and N. A. Wright, pp. 289–99. Springer, Berlin.

Nigro, N. D. and Campbell, R. L. (1978) Inhibition of azoxymethane-induced intestinal cancer by disulfiram. *Cancer Lett.*, **5**, 91–5.

Nigro, N. D., Bhadrachari, N. and Chomchai, C. (1973) A rat model for studying colonic cancer: effect of cholestyramine on induced tumours. *Dis. Colon Rectum*, **16**, 438–43.

Nigro, N. D., Sigh, D. V., Campbell, R. L. and Pak, M. S. (1975) Effect of dietary fat on intestinal tumours. *J. Natl. Cancer Inst.*, **54**, 439–42.

Nigro, N. D., Bull, A. W., Klopfer, B. A., *et al.* (1979) Effect of dietary fiber on azoxymethane-induced intestinal carcinogenesis in rats. *J. Natl. Cancer Inst.*, **77**, 269–76.

Nutter, R. L., Grindley, D. S., Kettering, J. D., Goude, A. G. and Slater, J. M. (1983) BALB/C mice fed milk or beef protein. *J. Natl. Cancer Inst.*, **71**, 867–75.

Nyman, M. and Asp, N.-G. (1982) Fermentation of dietary fibre components in the rat intestinal tract. *Br. J. Nutr.*, **47**, 357–64.

O'Brien, T. G., Simsiman, R. C. and Boutwell, R. K. (1975) Inducation of polyamine biosynthetic enzymes in mouse epidermis by tumour promoting agents. *Cancer Res.*, **35**, 1662–7.

O'Neill, I. K., Castegnaro, M., Brouet, I. and Povey, A. C. (1987) Magnetic semi-permeable polyethyleneimine microcapsules for monitoring of *N*-nitrosation in the gastrointestinal tract. *Carcinogenesis*, **8**, 1469–74.

O'Neill, I. K., Povey, A. C., Bingham, S., *et al.* (1988) Recoverable, semipermeable microencapsulated DNA surrogates for monitoring the colorectal cavity: in situ effects of fibre and meat in human diets or benzo[a]pyrene and possible endogenous cross-linking agents. In: *Methods for Detecting DNA Damaging*

Agents in Humans: Applications for Cancer Epidemiology and Prevention, ed. H. Bartch, K. Heminki and I. K. O'Neill, pp. 107–12. IARC.

Pence, B. and Buddingh, F. (1987) Inhibition of dietary fat promotion of colon carcinogenesis by supplemental calcium or vitamin D. *Proc. Am. Assoc. Cancer Res.*, **28**, 154.

Pence, B. C., Buddingh, F. and Yang, S. P. (1986) Multiple dietary factors in the enhancement of dimethylhydrazine carcinogenesis: main effect of indole-3-carbinol. *J. Natl. Cancer Inst.*, **62**, 1097–102.

Peng, R., Yong-Tu, Y. and Yang, C. S. (1982) The induction and competitive inhibition of high affinity microsomal nitrosodimethylamine demethylase by ethanol. *Carcinogenesis*, **3**, 1457–61.

Pollard, M. and Luckert, P. (1980) Indomethacin treatment of rats with dimethylhydrazine-induced intestinal tumours. *Cancer Treat. Rep.*, **64**, 1323–7.

Pollard, M. and Luckert, P. H. (1983) Prolonged antitumour effect of indomethacin on autochthonous intestinal tumours in rats. *J. Natl. Cancer Inst.*, **70**, 1103–5.

Pollard, M., Luckert, P. H. and Schmidt, M. A. (1983) The suppressive effect of piroxicam on autochthonous intestinal tumours in the rat. *Cancer Lett.*, **21**, 57–61.

Povey, A. C., Brouet, I., Bartch, H. and O'Neill, I. K. (1987) Building of benzo[a]pyrene metabolites in the rat intestinal lumen by magnetic polyethyleneimine microcapsules following an intragastric dose of [^{14}C]benzo[a]pyrene. *Carcinogenesis*, **8**, 825–31.

Raicht, R. F., Cohen, B. I., Fazzini, E. P., *et al.* (1980) Protective effect of plant sterols against chemically-induced colon tumours. *Cancer Res.*, **40**, 403–5.

Reddy, B. S. and Ohmori, T. (1981) Effect of intestinal microflora and dietary fat on 3,2′-dimethyl-4-aminobiphenyl-induced colon carcinogenesis in F344 rats. *Cancer Res.*, **41**, 1363–7.

Reddy, B. S. and Watanabe, K. (1979) Effect of cholesterol matabolites and promoting effect of lithocholic acid in colon carcinogenesis in germ-free and conventional F344 rats. *Cancer Res.*, **39**, 1521–4.

Reddy, B. S. and Wynder, E. L. (1977) Metabolic epidemiology of colon cancer: faecal bile acids and neutral sterols in colon cancer patients and patients with adenomatous polyps. *Cancer*, **39**, 2533–9.

Reddy, B. S., Weisburger, J. H., Narisawa, T. and Wynder E. L. (1974*a*) Colon carcinogenesis in germ-free rats with dimethylhydrazine and *N*-methyl-*N*-nitrosoguanidine. *Cancer Res.*, **34**, 2368–73.

Reddy, B. S., Weisburger, J. H. and Wynder, E. L. (1974*b*) Effects of dietary fat level and dimethylhydrazine on faecal acid and neutral sterol excretion and colon carcinogenesis in rats. *J. Natl. Cancer Inst.*, **52**, 507–11.

Reddy, B. S., Narisawa, T., Vukusich, D., Weisburger, J. H. and Wynder, E. L. (1976*a*) Effect of quality and quantity of dietary fat on dimethylhydrazine in colon carcinogenesis in rats. *Proc. Soc. Exp. Biol. Med.*, **151**, 237–9.

Reddy, B. S., Mastromarino, A., Gustafson, C., Lipkin, M. and Wynder, E. L. (1976*b*) Faecal bile acids and neutral sterols in patients with familial polyposis. *Cancer*, **38**, 1694–8.

Reddy, B. S., Mastromarino, A. and Gustafson, C., *et al.* (1976*c*) Faecal bile acids and neutral sterols in patients with familial polyposis coli. *Cancer*, **38**, 1694–8.

Reddy, B. S., Watanabe, K. and Weisburger, J. H. (1977*a*) Effect of high fat diet on colon carcinogenesis in F344 rats treated with 1,2-dimethylhydrazine, methylazoxymethanol acetate or methylnitrosourea. *Cancer Res.*, **37**, 4156–8.

Reddy, B. S., Watanabe, K., Weisburger, J. H. and Wynder, E. L. (1977*b*) Promoting effect of bile acids in colon carcinogenesis in germ free and conventional F344 rats. *Cancer Res.*, **37**, 3238–42.

Reddy, B. S., Martin, C. W. and Wynder, E. L. (1977*c*) Faecal bile acid and cholesterol metabolites of patients with ulcerative colitis: a high risk group for the development of colon cancer. *Cancer Res.*, **37**, 1697–701.

Reddy, B. S., Sharma, C. and Darby, L., *et al.* (1980) Metabolic epidemiology of large bowel cancer: faecal mutagens in high- and low-risk populations for colon cancer. *Mutat. Res.*, **72**, 511–22.

Reddy, B., Hirota, N. and Katayama, S. (1982) Effect of dietary sodium ascorbate on 1,2-dimethylhydrazine or methylnitrosourea-induced colon carcinogenesis in rats. *Carcinogenesis*, **3**, 1097–9.

Reddy, B. S., Maeura, Y. and Wayman, M. (1983) Effect of dietary corn bran and autohydrolysed lignin on 3,2-dimethyl-4-aminobiphenyl-induced intestinal carcinogenesis in male F344 rats. *J. Natl. Cancer Inst.*, **66**, 553–7.

Reddy, B. S., Wang, C. X. and Maruyama, H. (1987) Effect of restricted caloric intake on azoxymethane induced colon tumour incidence in male F344 rats. *Cancer Res.*, **47**, 1226–8.

Riddell, R. H. (1984) Dysplasia and cancer in ulcerative colitis: a soluble problem? *Scand. J. Gastroenterol.*, **19**, 137–49.

Rogers, A. E. and Newberne, P. M. (1980) Lipotope deficiency in experimental carcinogenesis. *Nutr. Cancer*, **2**, 104–112.

Rogers, K. J. and Pegg, A. E. (1977) Formation of *O*-6-methylguanine by alkylation of rat liver, colon and kidney DNA following administration of 1,2-dimethylhydrazine. *Cancer Res.*, **37**, 4082–7.

Romagnoli, P., Filipponi, F., Bandettini, L. and Bregnola, D. (1984) Increase of mitotic activity in the colonic mucosa of patients with colorectal cancer. *Dis. Colon Rectum*, **27**, 305–08.

Rozhin, J., Wilson, P. S., Bull, A. W. and Nigro, N. D. (1984) Ornithine decarboxylase activity in the rat and human colon cancer. *Cancer Res.*, **44**, 3226–30.

Sakata, T. and Yajima, T. (1984) Influence of short chain fatty acids on the epithelial cell division of the digestive tract. *Q. J. Exp. Physiol.*, **69**, 639–48.

Sarwal, A. N., Cohen, B. I. and Raicht, R. F., *et al.* (1979) Effects of dietary administration of chenodeoxycholic acid on *N*-methyl-*N*-nitrosourea-induced colon cancer in rats. *Biochim. Biophys. Acta*, **574**, 423–32.

Seitz, H. K. and Simanowski, U. A. (1988) Alcohol and carcinogenesis. *Annu. Rev. Nutrition*, **8**, 99–119.

Seitz, H. K., Czygan, P. and Waldnerr, R., *et al.* (1984) Enhancement of 1,2-dimethylhydrazine induced rectal carcinogenesis following chronic ethanol consumption in the rat. *Gastroenterology*, **86**, 886–91.

Seitz, H. K., Simanowski, U. A., Garzon, F. T. and Peters, T. J. (1987*a*) Alcohol and cancer. *Hepatology*, **7**, 816.

Seitz, H. K., Garzon, F. T., Simanowski, U. A. and Schmahl, D. (1987*b*) Erhote

Azetaldehydkonzentrationen als mögliche Ursache der tumor fordernden Wirkung von Alkohol im Rektum der Ratte. *Z. Gastroenterol.*, **8**, 551.

Shamsuddin, A. K. M. (1983) Comparative pathology: human large intestinal cancer and animal models. In: *Experimental Colon Carcinogenesis*, ed. H. Autrup and G. M. Williams, pp. 125–38. CRC Press, Boca Raton.

Silverman, J., Katayama, S. and Zelenakas, K., *et al.* (1981) Effect of reinoids on the induction of colon cancer in F344 rats by *N*-methyl-*N*-nitrosourea or by 1,2-dimethylhydrazine. *Carcinogenesis*, **2**, 1167–72.

Sjogren, H. O. and Steele, G. (1975) The immunology of large bowel carcinoma in a rat model. *Cancer*, **36**, 2469–71.

Sohn, O. S., Fiala, E. S., Puz, C., *et al.* (1987) Enhancement of rat liver microsomal metabolism of azoxymethane to methylazoxymethanol by chronic ethanol administration: similarity to the microsomal metabolism of *N*-nitrosomethylamine. *Cancer Res.*, **47**, 3123–9.

Soullier, B. K., Wilson, P. S. and Nigro, N. D. (1981) Effect of selenium on azoxymethane-induced intestinal cancer in rats fed a high fat diet. *Cancer Lett.*, **12**, 343–8.

Story, J. A. (1986) Modification of steroid excretion in response to dietary fibre. In: *Dietary Fibre: Basic and Clinical Aspects*, ed. G. V. Vahouny and D. Kritchevsky, pp. 253–64. Plenum Press, New York.

Subbish, R. (1971) Significance of dietary plant sterols in man and experimental animals. *Mayo Clin. Proc.*, **46**, 549–59.

Sugimura, T. (1985) Carcinogenicity of mutagenic heterocyclic amines formed during the cooking process. *Mutat. Res.*, **150**, 33–41.

Swenberg, J. A., Cooper, H. K., Buecheler, J. and Kleihues, P. (1979) 1,2-Dimethylhydrazine-induced methylation of DNA bases in various rat organs and the effect of pretreatment with disulfiram. *Cancer Res.*, **39**, 465–7.

Sych, F., Habs, M., and Schmahl, D. (1978) Chemotherapy studies in autochthonous rat tumours: intestinal cancer. *Z. Krebsforch*, **92**, 105–17.

Tanida, N., Sawada, K. and Kawaura, A., *et al.* (1989) Effects of oral administration of sulfolithocholic acid disodium salt and lithocholic acid disodium salt on *N*-methyl-*N*-nitrosourea-induced colonic tumourigenesis in conventional rats. *Cancer Res.*, **49**, 1178–81.

Teague, C. A. (1983) Morphological changes during chemical induction of colon cancer. In: *Experimental Colon Carcinogenesis*, ed. H. Autrup and G. M. Williams, pp. 107–24. CRC Press, Boca Raton.

Tibbetts, L. M., Chu, M. Y., Hager, J. C., *et al.* (1977) Chemotheraphy of cell line derived human colon carcinomas in mice immunosuppressed with antithymocyte serum. *Cancer*, **40**, 2651–5.

Toth, B. and Patil, K. (1982) Enhancing effect of vitamin E on murine intestinal tumourigenesis by 1,2-dimethylhydrazine dichloride. *J. Natl. Cancer Inst.*, **70**, 1107–11.

Tudek, B., Bird, R. P. and Bruce, W. R. (1985) Foci of aberrant crypts in the colons of mice and rats exposed to carcinogens associated with foods. *Cancer Res.*, **49**, 1236–40.

Tutton, R. P. J. M. and Barkla, D. H. (1983) Regulation of cell kinetics and colon cancer. In: *Experimental Colon Carcinogenesis*, ed. H. Autrup and G. M. Williams, pp. 199–214. CRC Press, Boca Raton.

Visek, W. J. and Clinton, S. K. (1983) Dietary fat and breast cancer. In: *Dietary Fats and Health*, ed. E. G. Perkins and W. J. Viset, pp. 721–8. American Oil Society, Champaign.

Ward, J. M., Yamamoto, R. S. and Brown C. A. (1973) Pathology of intestinal neoplasms and other lesions in rats exposed to azoxymethane. *J. Natl. Cancer Inst.*, **51**, 1029–39.

Wargovich, M. J. (1987). Diallyl sulfide, a flavour component of garlic (*Allium sativum*) inhibits dimethylhydrazine-induced colon cancer. *Carcinogenesis*, **8**, 1239–41.

Watanabe, K., Reddy, B. S., Wong, C. Q. and Weisburger, J. H. (1978*a*) Effect of dietary alfalfa, pectin and wheat bran on azoxymethane- or methyl nitrosourea-induced colon carcinogenesis in F344 rats. *J. Natl. Cancer Inst.*, **63**, 141–5.

Watanabe, K., Reddy, B. S., Wong, Q. C. and Weisburger, J. H. (1978*b*) Effect of dietary undegraded carageenan on colon carcinogenesis in F344 rats treated with azoxymethane or methylnitrosourea. *Cancer Res.*, **38**, 4427–30.

Wattenberg, L. W. (1984) Inhibition of carcinogen-induced neoplasia by sodium cyanate, tert-butyl isocyanate and benzyl isothiocyanate administered subsequent to carcinogen exposure. *Cancer Res.*, **41**, 2991–4.

Wattenberg, L. W. (1985) Chemoprevention of cancer. *Cancer Res.*, **45**, 1–8.

Weed, H. G., McGandy, R. B. and Kennedy, A. R. (1985) Protection against dimethylhydrazine-induced adenomatous tumours of the mouse colon by the dietary addition of an extract of soybeans containing the Bowman–Birk protease inhibitor. *Carcinogenesis*, **8**, 1239–41.

Weisburger, J. H. (1989) Dietary prevention of colorectal cancer. In: *Colorectal Cancer*, ed. H. K. Seitz *et al.*, pp. 361–74. Springer, Berlin.

Weisburger, J. H. and Fiala, E. S. (1983) Experimental colon carcinogens and their mode of action. In: *Experimental Colon Carcinogenesis*, ed. H. Autrup and G. M. Williams, pp. 27–50. CRC Press, Boca Raton.

Weisburger, E. K., Evarts, R. P. and Wenk, M. L. (1977) Inhibitory effect of butylated hydroxytoluene (BHT) on intestinal carcinogenesis in rats induced by azoxymethane. *Food Cosmet. Toxicol.*, **15**, 139–41.

Williamson, R. C. N. and Rainey, J. R. (1984) The relationship between intestinal hyperplasia and carcinogenesis. *Scand. J. Gastroenterol.*, **19**, 57–76.

Williamson, R. C. N., Bauer, F., Terpstra, O., Ross, J. S. and Malt, R. A. (1980) Contrasting effects of subtotal enteric bypass, enterectomy and colectomy on azoxymethane-induced intestinal carcinogenesis. *Cancer Res.*, **40**, 538–43.

Wilson, R. B., Hutcheson, D. P. and Wideman, L. (1977) Dimethylhydrazine-induced colon tumours in rats fed diets containing beef fat or corn oil with and without wheat bran. *Am. J. Clin. Nutr.*, **30**, 176–81.

Wright, N. and Alison, M. (1984) *The Biology of Epithelial Cell Populations*. Clarendon Press, Oxford.

Yuspa, S. H., Lichti, U., Ben, T., *et al.* (1976) Phorbol ester tumour promoters stimulate DNA synthesis and ornithine decarboxylase activity in mouse epidermal cell cultures. *Nature*, **262**, 402–4.

Zeller, J. and Beiger, M. R. (1984) Chemically-induced autochthonous tumour models in experimental chemotherapy. *Behring Inst. Mitt.*, **74**, 201–8.

5

In vitro studies

Current theories of carcinogenesis based on experimental systems suggest that carcinogenesis may be divided into the steps of 'initiation', 'promotion' (at least two steps) and progression. For human colorectal carcinoma at least four or five distinct genetic stages have been identified (Fearon and Vogelstein, 1990).

Colorectal tumours have provided and will continue to provide an excellent system in which to search for and study the genetic alterations involved in the development of human neoplasias. Firstly, samples representing the various stages of development through the adenoma–carcinoma sequence can be obtained for the direct study of cellular transforming genes, DNA ploidy and cytogenetics. Cell lines can be established from biopsy samples and the adenoma–carcinoma sequence can now be mimicked in a colorectal cell line in culture (Williams *et al.*, 1990). Moreover, the availability of biopsy samples from individuals with an inherited predisposition to the tumour has facilitated many studies in search of the properties that might be involved in increased susceptibility. Also, standard non-colorectal *in vitro* cell systems have facilitated the identification of some of the environmental or dietary factors involved in the aetiology of the disease.

Studies on cell cultures established from individuals with an inherited predisposition to colorectal carcinoma

Although many colorectal carcinoma cell lines exist (Carrel *et al.*, 1976; Liebovitz *et al.*, 1976; Brattain *et al.*, 1983; Namba *et al.*, 1983; Danes, 1985), it is really cell lines established from individuals with an inherited predisposition to colorectal carcinoma such as FPC (FAP) that are the most appropriate for the study of the cellular and molecular events involved in the progression of adenomas or pre-malignant cells to carcinoma cells. Most of the early cell culture studies were performed on skin fibroblasts from patients with FPC (FAP), the thesis being that these representative somatic cells from individuals with an inherited predisposition to colorectal cancer might carry a mutation analogous to the 'initiation' event of multistage carcinogenesis (Kinsella and Gainer, 1984; Gainer *et al.*, 1984). Skin fibroblasts were chosen because of the relative ease with which they could be obtained (minimal distress to the patient) and because of the relative ease with which they could be grown. Skin fibroblasts also provide the opportunity to investigate a single cell type under reproducible conditions.

Investigation of the properties of these cells which might render them more susceptible to malignant transformation *in vivo* included chromosomal instability, sensitivity to carcinogenic agents, susceptibility to transformation and mutation by a variety of agents, and differences in phenotypic properties.

Growth and phenotypic properties of skin fibroblasts from affected individuals

The unusual growth properties and increased transformability of skin fibroblasts from affected individuals were first shown by Pfeffer *et al.* (1976) and Pfeffer and Kopelovich (1977). Kopelovich and Sirlin (1980) reported T-antigen display and transformation following infection with simian virus 40 (SV40) in apparently karyologically normal cells. Rasheed and Gardner (1981), however, reported skin fibroblasts from FPC (FAP) patients, Gardner's syndrome (GS) patients and asymptomatic family members to be morphologically normal and to have growth rates similar to untreated 'normal' controls. However, cells from FPC (FAP) and GS patients could generally be distinguished from normal cells by their increased growth properties, i.e. their plating efficiency and saturation density in low serum was several-fold greater than for normal cells. By far the most striking difference observed, though, was the susceptibility of cells from FPC (FAP) and GS patients to transformation by Kirsten murine sarcoma virus. (Ki-MuSV) (Pfeffer and Kopelovich, 1977; Rasheed and Gardner, 1981). This is particularly interesting in view of the fact that mutations at codon 12 and rarely codon 61 in the normal cellular homologue of the Ki-MuSV gene, Ki-*ras*, are to be found at high frequency (up to 50 per cent) in colorectal tumours (Bos *et al.*, 1987; Forrester *et al.*, 1987).

In vitro *transformation*

On the basis of the assumption that somatic cells from individuals with an inherited predisposition to cancer might be at least one step further along the multistep pathway to malignancy than a normal cell, studies were initiated to investigate their susceptibility to malignant transformation. Pfeffer and Kopelovich (1977) reported that cultured skin fibroblasts from FPC (FAP) individuals were especially susceptible to morphological transformation by the Kirsten murine sarcoma virus (Ki-MuSV). This was confirmed by Rasheed and Gardner (1981), who demonstrated that skin fibroblasts from FPC (FAP) patients could be transformed with 100- to 1000-fold the efficiency of normal cells. Similarly, morphological transformation by the hybrid virus Adeno12–SV40 took 2 weeks in skin fibroblasts from FPC (FAP) patients and 1–2 months in cells from normal individuals. Such differences in susceptibility to viral transformation clearly separated those individuals with an inherited predisposition to cancer from the normal controls and therefore was postulated as an assay for cancer susceptibility. Increased genetic susceptibility of human skin fibroblasts to SV40 infection had also been suggested by Todaro and others (Todaro *et al.*, 1966; Todaro, 1968; Miller and Todaro, 1969) to be an indicator of cancer risk. Kopelovich and Sirlin (1980) reported an increased sensitivity to T-antigen display and morphologically transformed focus production of karyologically normal skin fibroblasts from FPC (FAP) individuals. However, none of these SV40-transformed cells were immortal or produced tumours in nude mice.

Skin fibroblasts from FPC (FAP) patients were also reported to be more susceptible to morphological transformation by the chemical carcinogen *N*-methyl-*N′*-nitro-*N*-nitrosoguanidine (MNNG) (Rhim *et al.*, 1980). The resultant cells exhibited anchorage-independent growth on agar, a prolonged lifespan in culture and a marked increase in cell ploidy when compared with untreated cells (Rhim *et al.*, 1980). Cells from FPC (FAP) individuals, but not their age-matched controls, have been transformed by γ-irradiation to anchorage-independent growth (Kopelovich *et al.*, 1981). Skin fibroblasts from patients with FPC (FAP) have also been reported to be susceptible to transformation by the tumour promoter TPA(12-*O*-tetradecanoylphorbol-13-acetate) alone (Kopelovich *et al.*, 1979; Gainer *et al.*, 1984). TPA treatment of FPC (FAP) skin fibroblasts (Kopelovich *et al.*, 1979) resulted in anchorage-independent cells that grew on agar and cells that produced tumours when injected into the immune-privileged site in the anterior chamber of the nude mouse eye. No tumours were obtained when the cells were injected subcutaneously into nude mice; also there was no strict correlation between the ability to form tumours and anchorage independence. These observations were for the most part confirmed by Gainer *et al.* (1984) and Kinsella and Gainer (1984), who reported low-frequency anchorage-independent growth on methylcellulose following continuous exposure to the tumour promoter TPA. None of the anchorage-independent cell lines produced tumours in nude mice following subcutaneous injection. Parallel cytogenetic analyses showed TPA to increase not only tetraploidy but also the chromosome aberration frequency, with several quadriradial chromosomes being observed in the tetraploid cells. In contrast Rasheed and Gardner (1981) and Antecol and Mukherjee (1982) failed to see transformation of any kind with TPA.

Overall, the inability of the TPA-treated FPC (FAP) cells to grow reproducibly on agar or methylcellulose or to produce tumours when injected subcutaneously into nude mice suggests that such cells are really only partially transformed. Moreover, none of the viral, chemical or physical agents cited above or the introduction of an N-*ras* oncogene cDNA (Kinsella, unpublished observations) were able to induce transformation to a malignant phenotype, which suggests that other steps are required. The general feeling, however, is that skin fibroblast cells from individuals with FPC (FAP) are more susceptible to transforming agents than normal skin fibroblasts (Kinsella, 1988).

The only true study of *in vitro* transformation with direct relevance to colorectal cancer is that of Williams *et al.* (1990) involving the transformation of the pre-malignant epithelial colonic adenoma cell line. This cell line was derived from a 3–4 cm mildly dysplastic tubular adenoma from a patient with FPC (FAP) (Pareskeva *et al.*, 1984). A rare aneuploid clonogenic variant was isolated from the diploid parent cell line and treated with sodium butyrate. This gave rise to a cell line that had an increased cloning efficiency (CE) on plastic but remained anchorage-dependent and non-tumourigenic. After exposure of these cells to MNNG, an anchorage-independent cell line was isolated which on continuous *in vitro* passage became tumourigenic in nude mice and was characterised by specific chromosomal changes. This is the first example of the malignant progression of human colonic epithelial cells *in vitro* and confirms the complex multistep nature of the process as studied *in vivo* (Vogelstein *et al.*, 1988; Fearon and Vogelstein, 1990).

Cytogenetic analysis

Cytogenetic analysis has shown that most cancers are chromosomally abnormal and chromosomal instability has been identified in a variety of so-called cancer-prone or cancer predisposing syndromes such as Bloom's syndrome (German, 1974), Fanconi's anaemia (Schroeder and Kurth, 1971; Schroeder and German, 1974) and ataxia telangiectasia (Saadi *et al.*, 1980). It was not unreasonable, therefore, to suppose that chromosomal instability might also be a property of cells from individuals with an inherited predisposition to colorectal carcinoma.

Hori *et al.* (1980) reported that the spontaneous levels of chromatid and chromosome aberrations were the same for skin fibroblasts from FPC (FAP) patients as they were for cells from normal individuals. However, in the same study skin fibroblasts from individuals with FPC (FAP) treated with MNNG showed elevated chromosomal instability when compared with controls. More recently, though, a general chromosomal instability has been noted in a range of somatic cells from polyposis patients (Gardner *et al.*, 1982; Delhanty *et al.*, 1983). Gardner *et al.* (1982) noted excessive aneuploidy, tetraploidy and structural aberrations in skin fibroblasts and lymphocytes from affected individuals. Delhanty *et al.* (1983) observed chromosomal instability in lymphocytes, colonic epithelial cells, colonic fibroblasts and skin fibroblasts which was associated with occasional high levels of tetraploidy. Since increased chromosome breakage and rearrangement appeared to be a property of all the tissues examined the authors suggested that FPC (FAP) might in fact be a chromosome breakage syndrome. Certainly in this study all classes of abnormality were increased in the skin fibroblasts from polyposis patients. The high number of clonally abnormal cells as early as passage 2 or 3 was the most striking feature. The fact that the clone could represent 80–100 per cent of the cells at such an early stage suggested either the presence of such changes *in vivo* or a strong proliferative advantage *in vitro*.

Heim *et al.* (1984), in a study of spontaneous and MNNG-induced chromatid and iso-chromatid breaks and interchanges in skin fibroblasts from patients with FPC (FAP) and from unaffected healthy members of the FPC (FAP) families, showed both categories of aberration (spontaneous and induced) to be elevated approximately 2-fold in the cells from FPC (FAP) patients. However, a study by the same author in lymphocytes (Heim, 1985) showed that although both spontaneous and mitomycin-C-induced aberrations were higher in the patients than the controls, the difference was not statistically significant. More recently, chromosomal analysis using high-resolution G-banding of lymphocytes from individuals with inherited non-polyposis colon cancer syndrome failed to identify any structural chromosome abnormalities or any difference in mitomycin-C-induced sister chromatid exchanges (SCEs) between the cells of affected individuals and controls (Lukeis *et al.*, 1987). Previous studies of SCE levels in patients with FPC (FAP) had also failed to reveal diagnostic or other differences (Gardner *et al.*, 1985).

Cytogenetic studies also suggested that increased tetraploidy might be a feature of the cultured cells from FPC (FAP) patients (Danes, 1981;

Delhanty *et al.*, 1983) which could be exploited as a possible biomarker for genetic predisposition to colorectal carcinoma. In the studies of Delhanty *et al.* (1983), colonic epithelial-like cultures on the whole showed remarkably low tetraploidy. Whilst tetraploid levels in colon fibroblast cultures established from the same tissue specimen were extremely variable, none of the patients showing high tetraploidy in their colon fibroblasts showed high tetraploidy in their skin fibroblasts. Repeat biopsies from two patients who originally showed increased tetraploidy, failed to produce similarly high levels. However, clonal rearrangements were present in both of the second biopsy cultures. These findings suggested that the high levels of tetraploidy found in the initial cultures might be another manifestation of clone formation. *In vitro* tetraploidy (IVT) has been identified in skin fibroblasts from heritable colon cancer families (Danes, 1976, 1981; Danes and Alm, 1981; Svendsen *et al.*, 1989) as well as those from non-heritable colon cancer families (Svendsen *et al.*, 1985, 1987). In fact, IVT in human skin fibroblasts was proposed as an assay for the identification of cancer genotypes (Danes *et al.*, 1986). No correlation was found for IVT with skin fibroblasts from patients with ulcerative colitis (Svendsen *et al.*, 1987*b*). These data therefore support the thesis of Wolman (1985) that elevated levels of intrinsic chromosome breakage and numerical chromosomal instability increase the probability of the evolution of a chromosomally aberrant population of cells with a cellular growth advantage.

Chromosomal analysis of adenomas and carcinomas

Cytogenetic analysis of colon cancer families has until recently been concentrated on the skin fibroblasts and lymphocytes from 'affected' individuals (see above), with a view to identifying some constitutive chromosomal instability. Progressive chromosomal changes have been studied in a variety of tumour cell lines established from FPC (FAP) and inherited non-polyposis colon cancer patients (Namba *et al.*, 1983; Paraskeva *et al.*, 1989 *a*, *b*; Jenkyn *et al.*, 1987) or human xenografts in nude mice (Lothe *et al.*, 1987). However, at best the reports of chromosomal changes in colorectal cancer are confusing.

Cytogenetic analysis of 18 fresh tumour specimens in the near-diploid range (Muleris *et al.* 1987) demonstrated no numerical chromosome abnormalities for chromosomes 1, 2, 6, 10, 11, 17, 19 or 21. All other chromosomes were involved in losses or gains at varying frequencies. The most frequent loss was clearly chromosome 18 (12/18 cases). The next was chromosome 14 (5/18 cases), then chromosome 4 (4/18 cases) and then chromsome 15 (3/18 cases). All the tumours had structural rearrangements with chromosome 17, the chromosome most frequently involved in marker formation with the concomitant loss of the short arm (16/18 cases). The consistency of the numerical changes in this study and a previous one from the same group (Muleris *et al.*, 1985) suggested a characteristic chromosomal pattern for colorectal carcinoma.

Direct cytogenetic analysis of cells of a sessile benign tubulo-villous adenoma (Couturier-Turpin *et al.*, 1988) showed chromosome 18 to be missing in 80 per cent of cells. A marker for chromosome 1 was observed in 58 per cent of cells and the loss of chromosome 17 in 5 out of 13 cells examined. Chromosome 5, that bears the gene for FPC (FAP) implicated in 20 per cent of common colorectal cancers (Solomon *et al.*, 1987), was missing in only 2 out of 13 cells. None of the cells examined in this study were chromosomally normal, with 77 per cent of cells having more than the normal number of chromosomes. This demonstration of significant cytogenetic abnormalities in an apparently benign adenoma was surprising because according to theories of the clonal evolution of cancer as applied to the adenoma–carcinoma sequence, adenomas should really only show limited cytogenetic abnormalities. The similarity in the chromosome aberrations of the adenoma with those of the carcinomas described previously, suggests that the adenoma has already undergone transformation.

Similar chromosome abnormalities were also observed when direct cytogenetic analysis was performed on an FPC (FAP) tumour biopsy (Muleris *et al.*, 1989). The stem line had 45 chromosomes, with several clonal chromosome aberrations of which an unbalanced rearrangement of chromosome 17 leading to a loss of its short (p) arm and a loss of chromosome 18 were the most common. High-resolution cytogenetic analysis of the blood lymphocytes from the same patient did not reveal any constitutive chromosome abnormality. None of the cells had deletions of the long (q) arm of chromosome 5. So, once again the cytogenetic findings for FPC (FAP) were similar to those for the spontaneous colorectal carcinoma reported above (Muleris *et al.*, 1989).

The evidence from these cytogenetic studies therefore quite strongly implicates the loss of specific chromosomal regions in the development of colorectal neoplasia, namely chromosome 17p and chromsome 18q. In fact Monpezat *et al.* (1988), from studies of polyploid carcinomas, suggested that many colorectal carcinomas arose from a single cell that has lost part of either chromosome 17 or 18 or both. Such allelic losses can in turn be interpreted as evidence that these specific regions of the chromosome contain suppressor genes. The loss of a large portion of chromosome 17p through chromosome loss or mitotic recombination has been confirmed using polymorphic probes in more than 75 per cent of colorectal carcinomas (Vogelstein *et al.*, 1988; Delattre *et al.*, 1989; Fearon and Vogelstein, 1990). Moreover these allelic losses were found to be associated with the progression from adenoma to carcinoma (Fearon *et al.*, 1987; Vogelstein *et al.*, 1988) and to be relatively infrequent in adenomas at any stage (Fig. 5.1; Fearon and Vogelstein, 1990).

The region of chromosome 17 loss common to colorectal tumours has been identified as that containing the p53 gene (Baker *et al.*, 1989). Mutations resulting in amino acid substitutions in the p53 gene product have frequently been found to occur concomitantly with the loss of the remaining wild-type allele as a result of the deletion of the p arm of the other chromosome 17 (Baker *et al.*, 1989; Nigro *et al.*, 1989). These data coupled with those from *in vitro* transformation systems suggest that the wild-type p53 gene functions as a tumour suppressor gene (Eliyahu *et al.*, 1989; Finlay *et al.*, 1989). Allelic loss of chromosome 18q has also been confirmed in 70 per cent of carcinomas and in almost 50 per cent of late adenomas (Vogelstein *et al.*, 1988). The common region of allelic loss has been identified as another candidate for a suppressor gene (Fearon *et al.*, 1990). The gene, DCC (deleted in colon cancer), which encodes a protein related to the family of adhesion molecules, is expressed in normal colonic

Fig. 5.1. Frequency of *ras* gene mutations and chromosome 17p deletions in colorectal tumours. Early stage adenomas were those 1 cm in size or less. Intermediate stage adenomas were greater than 1 cm in size but did not contain foci of adenoma. Late stage carcinomas were greater than 1 cm in size and contained foci of carcinomas (Fearon and Vogelstein, 1990).

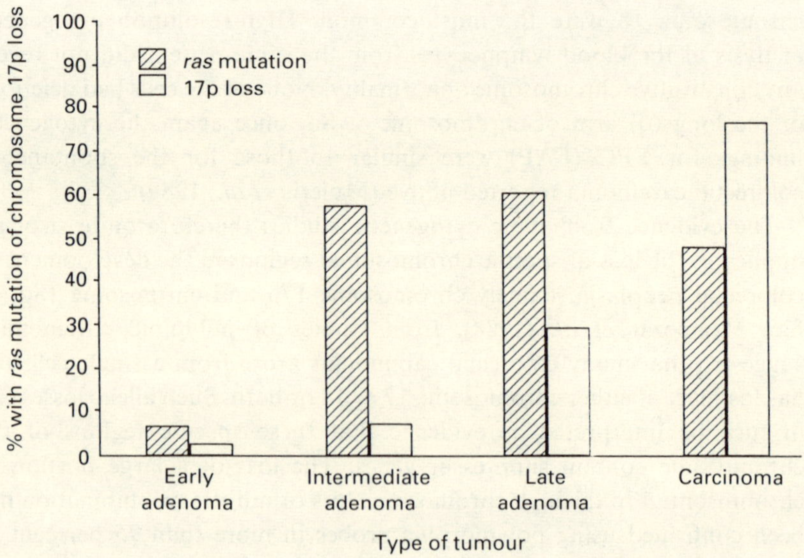

mucosa but its expression is reduced or absent in the majority of colorectal carcinomas.

Syndromes which predispose to cancer, such as FPC (FAP) in the case of colorectal cancer, are thought to result from a germ-line inactivation of one copy of a tumour suppressor gene. However, for colorectal disease, the cytogenetic studies above and the studies of allelic loss in adenomas from FPC (FAP) patients (Solomon *et al.*, 1987; Vogelstein *et al.*, 1988; Sasaki *et al.*, 1989) have not revealed loss of the chromosome region linked to this syndrome. This can be explained if some suppressor gene mutations affect growth even in the presence of a wild-type allele. Wildrick and Boman (1988), however, using DNA pairs from colon cancer patients reported 5q loss in 27 per cent of tumours.

Volgelstein's group also addressed the problem of the other chromosome losses observed in the classical cytogenetic studies of tumours. Polymorphic markers from every non-acrocentric autosomal arm were studied in colorectal carcinomas and regions of chromosomes 1q, 4p, 6p, 6q, 8p, 9q and 22q, were lost in 25–50 per cent of cases studied (Fig. 5.2). The 8p loss was in complete contrast to the familial 8q22 deletion found in all cells of a colon tumour by Shabtai *et al.* (1988) and the results of a study of rectosigmoidal carcinomas by Ferti *et al.* (1988) which again implicated 8q. Other chromosome losses were also observed. Overall, the median number of allelic losses per tumour was four or five and patients with more than the median number of allelic losses in their tumours had a considerably worse prognosis (Kern *et al.*, 1989; Vogelstein *et al.*, 1989). This was irrespective of other clinical indicators.

Thus the thesis was and is (Fearon and Vogelstein, 1990) that the allelic losses observed in colorectal carcinomas (Fig. 5.2) are representative of two processes. Firstly, the chromosomal regions lost in the majority of colorectal cancers such as those on 17p and 18q presumably contain suppressor genes, whilst one explanation of the additional allelic losses might be that there are many tumour suppressor genes throughout the genome (reviewed by Ponder, 1988; Sager, 1989). The observed heterogeneity in the biological properties of colorectal tumours from different patients is presumably a consequence of the heterogeneity of the allelic loss in different tumours. It has recently been hypothesised that the end-to-end chromosome fusions observed in some tumours could play a role in the genetic instability associated with tumourigenesis. Hastie *et al.* (1990), demonstrated that in most of the colorectal carcinomas analysed there was a reduction in the length of the G-rich telomeric region at the ends of the chromosomes when compared with chromosomes from the normal colonic mucosae from the same patients. Hastie *et al.* (1990) proposed that telomere reduction and loss could contribute to the genetic instability of these tumours by virtue of the fact that chromosomes lacking terminal repeats may be less stable and be lost at a higher frequency. Alternatively, chromosomes without telomeres may be prone to fusion-bridge breakage such that daughter cells can receive partly deleted and partly duplicated chromosomes respectively. Chromosome deletions or losses by these routes could play a part in generating the allele losses that occur in colorectal carcinomas (Vogelstein *et al.*, 1988; Fearon and Vogelstein, 1990). Some of the allele losses occur at the adenoma stage, but the majority are not apparent until the carcinoma stage. The telomere reductions, however, are already seen at the adenoma stage, suggesting that these changes could be involved in causing the chromosome rearrangements that are subsequently observed in the carcinoma.

Studies of cell lines established from colon carcinomas and adenomas presented a completely different chromosomal bias. A colon carcinoma cell line established from a metastatic lymph node of a patient with FPC (FAP) had an essentially diploid chromosome number, but all the karyotypes examined were abnormal with 7p+ and +13, accompanied by loss of chromosome 19 or 20 (Namba *et al.*, 1983). Jenkyn *et al.* (1987) reported a trisomy 1q in a colon carcinoma cell line from a patient with inherited non-polyposis colorectal cancer, whilst an epithelial cell line established from a sporadic villous adenoma exhibited a deletion of chromsome 1 and was monosomic for chromosome 18 (Pareskeva *et al.*,

Fig. 5.2. Frequency of allelic deletions in individual chromosomes in colorectal carcinomas (Fearon and Vogelstein, 1990).

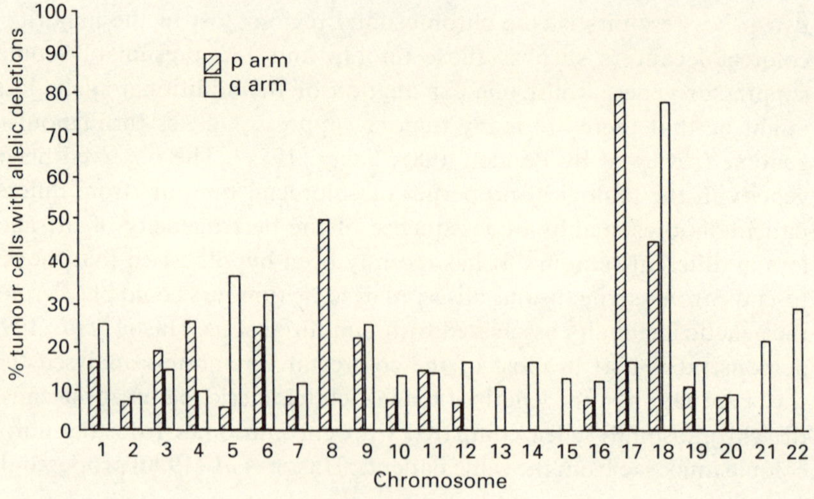

1989*a*). A possible chromosome 1 involvement in colorectal cancer had been reported previously by Kovacs (1978) and Richmann *et al.* (1984). An epithelial cell line established from a sporadic tubular adenoma had only one normal copy of chromosomes 6, 7, 14, 18 and 22 and had several marker chromosomes (Pareskeva *et al.*, 1989*a*). Neither of these cell lines was tumourigenic, so in neither case were the cytogenetic abnormalities sufficient for tumourigenesis. Both cell lines, however, were monosomic for chromosome 18, confirming the *in vivo* observation that this is a key step in colorectal tumour progression. Another epithelial cell line derived from a tubular adenoma from an FPC (FAP) patient had an isochromosome 1q associated with *in vitro* immortalisation (Pareskeva *et al.*, 1989*b*). Following selection *in vitro* and treatment with MNNG it progressed to malignancy and a karyotype that included 1–2 copies of an abnormal chromosome 1, which had undergone a complex rearrangement, as well as 1–2 copies of a normal chromosome 1, up to six copies of chromosomes 7, 9 and 13, and monosomy of chromosome 18 (Williams *et al.*, 1990). This study represents the first evidence for the adenoma–carcinoma sequence *in vitro*.

DNA ploidy studies

Alterations in ploidy levels are a well-recognised feature of human solid tumours, with a range of aneuploidy of from 50 to 90 per cent (Friedlander *et al.*, 1984). Analysis of the DNA content of colorectal tumours, using for the most part flow cytometric analysis of propidium iodide labelled cells, appeared to offer good prognostic information in early studies. Wolley *et al.* (1982) provided the first prospective report on the prognostic value of DNA content for colorectal tumours. In their study patients with aneuploid tumours had a poor prognosis. This observation was supported by the studies of Armitage *et al.* (1985) on paraffin-embedded material from 134 carcinomas, and those of Emdin *et al.* (1987) on 37 fresh specimens from the caecum, colon and rectum. DNA analysis of these specimens showed 62 per cent to be aneuploid, the aneuploidy being associated with advanced Dukes' C tumours, but with an equal distribution of aneuploid and diploid tumours in Dukes' A and B. Schutte *et al.* (1987) evaluated the prognostic significance of tumour DNA content in a large series of large bowel carcinomas in a prospective randomised surgical trial. Flow cytometric analysis was performed on tissue taken from 279 paraffin blocks and showed a characteristic bimodal distribution of aneuploidy with tumours having either a near-diploid or a triploid-tetraploid mode. In this study the degree of aneuploidy was not significantly correlated with survival, but Dukes' C cases showed a statistically significant association between tumour ploidy and overall survival.

Forslund *et al.* (1984) conducted a retrospective study on rectal carcinomas in 25 patients using cytophotometric measurements on stained histological sections and were able to show that aneuploid tumours had a worse prognosis. Kokal *et al.* (1986), however, demonstrated that DNA content was only an important prognostic indicator in patients with primary disease. In patients with hepatic metastases, the DNA content of the metastases bore no relationship to the patients' survival or their response to therapy. A retrospective flow cytometric study was also undertaken to investigate the origin of multiple, synchronous, apparently primary carcinomas of the colon in ten patients. In three out of the ten cases, the tumours within each colon differed with respect to DNA ploidy, in four cases all the tumours were diploid and in three cases both tumours within each colon had identical aneuploid indices. These replicate aneuploid indices strongly suggested a common origin for the multiple tumours in these patients. The tumours in the two other groups were compatible with either single or multiple origins. The data therefore support the thesis that at least in some cases primary colon carcinomas may arise as transluminal metastases from a single lesion.

In view of the adenoma–carcinoma sequence ploidy studies were also conducted on adenomatous polyps of the colon. Whitehead *et al.* (1985), using cytophotometric measurements, showed all 16 adenomatous polyps examined to be diploid, even those with severe dysplasia. This, coupled with the fact that some carcinomas are diploid, suggests that the ploidy abnormalities associated with some carcinomas occur some time after invasion has occurred. Hamada *et al.* (1987) failed to find polyploid or aneuploid cells in 52 adenomas, irrespective of their proliferative capacity or whether they were located adjacent to a carcinoma. However, Scott *et al.* (1987*a*) in a flow cytometric study of 21 adenomas from high-risk patients who had a resection for invasive carcinoma sometime after polypectomy, showed three (13 per cent) to be aneuploid. All three aneuploid polyps were found in the distal colon and two were greater than 2 cm in size. This tendency for DNA aneuploidy in larger polyps had been reported previously by Quirke *et al.* (1986) and van den Ingh *et al.* (1985), whilst Goh and Jass (1986) found a significant trend between severity of adenoma dysplasia and the occurrence of DNA aneuploidy.

Overall, however, the relatively low incidence of DNA aneuploidy in adenomas compared with carcinomas probably reflects the long natural history of the adenoma–carcinoma sequence, i.e. an average of 10–15 years for progression from one to the other (Morson, 1974). Isolated versus cancer-associated adenomas revealed no increased incidence of DNA aneuploidy. It can be concluded, therefore, that the use of DNA content measurements of aneuploidy in adenomas does not identify patients at risk from the adenoma–carcinoma sequence. However, in one prospective flow cytometric study, aneuploidy was detected in 9 per cent of patients with long-standing ulcerative colitis associated with dysplasia and was considered helpful, when coupled with histopathological investigations, for the detection of potential malignancy in this disease (Lofberg *et al.*, 1987). In another study, adenomas from seven out of nine patients with a family history exhibited DNA aneuploidy (Sciallero *et al.*, 1988).

This test, therefore, although carefully controlled (Petersen and Friedrich, 1986; Scott *et al.*, 1987*b*) is still controversial. Jones *et al.* (1988) suggested that conflicting results may have arisen due to differences in patient selection, techniques and data interpretation. DNA aneuploidy is defined as the presence of at least two separate G_0/G_1 peaks (Hiddemann *et al.*, 1984), but the minimum size of the peak considered to constitute aneuploidy varies amongst investigators. DNA aneuploid histograms also vary such that there may be identifiable sub-groups within them, which would more accurately predict prognosis. A survival advantage has already been suggested for patients with tetraploid DNA tumours (Quirke *et al.*, 1987). Therefore the feeling is that if the determination of DNA ploidy by, for example, flow cytometry, is to have any clinical application then the definitions of DNA aneuploidy and subaneuploidy will have to be standardised.

Differential response of normal, pre-malignant and malignant colonic epithelial cells to the tumour promoter TPA and selective endogenous mitogens

Patients with an inherited predisposition to colon cancer are known to exhibit differences within the colonic crypt in the distribution of their DNA synthesising cells when compared with individuals from cancer-free families (Deschner and Lipkin, 1975; Lipkin, 1974; Iwana *et al.*, 1977; Lipkin *et al.*, 1983). Also, *in vitro* the tumour promoter TPA (12-*O*-tetradecanoylphorbol-13-acetate) has been shown to increase DNA synthesis on average 8-fold in cultured colonic epithelial cells from five out of six FPC (FAP) patients (Friedman *et al.*, 1984*a*). No such stimulation of DNA synthesis was observed in cultures of colonic epithelial cells from 13 non-polyposis patients at high risk of developing colon carcinoma, or in cells from five low-risk individuals. Fibroblasts from FPC (FAP) individuals were already known to be more resistant to the toxic effects of TPA than normal fibroblasts (Kopelovich, 1981) and TPA had been reported to induce a mitogenic response in four tubular adenomas (Friedman *et al.*, 1981). Thus, the authors concluded that FPC (FAP) cells were the precursors of tubular adenomas and that their progression from a benign to a more advanced pre-malignant stage might be influenced by endogenous tumour promoters.

Moreover, in a separate study the same authors showed that the induction of plasminogen activator (PA) by TPA could be used to order histologically distinct classes of human colonic adenomas in primary culture (Friedman *et al.*, 1984*b*). Histopathologically the most benign tumours were the small, pure tubular adenomas without dysplasia. Six out of seven of these failed to secrete PA in response to TPA. Consistent with this, colonic epithelial cells from FPC (FAP) patients failed to respond to TPA by secreting PA even though their proliferative fraction is increased. TPA treatment of two cultured villous adenomas, one with infiltrating carcinoma and one with a focus of moderately dysplastic cells, showed only a small subpopulation to respond by PA secretion. This pattern of secretion was confirmed by screening additional villous, tubulo-villous and tubular adenomas. In 23 out of 24 cases, the presence of dysplastic subpopulations of cells correlated with PA secretion. Seven out of seven carcinomas secreted PA in response to TPA. The authors concluded, therefore, that the tumour cells had the ability to respond to TPA by secreting PA. The subpopulation of villous cells which secreted PA in the absence of dysplasia (three cases) provided evidence of a tumour evolution in which such villous populations were the first pre-malignant cell types to acquire PA-associated TPA responsiveness. The tubular adenoma cells were not at an advanced enough pre-malignant stage to respond.

Thus, it seemed that the genetic changes which made colon cells pre-malignant also directly or indirectly conferred susceptibility to tumour promoters such as TPA. TPA did not induce proliferation of normal cells (Friedman *et al.*, 1984*a*), but did induce proliferation of pre-malignant cells from patients with FPC (FAP) and proliferation of tubular adenomas. The receptor for TPA is protein kinase C, which is activated within the cell by diacylglycerol. Friedman *et al.* (1989) demonstrated the presence of diglycerides in faecal extracts at concentrations which induced the mitogenesis of adenoma and carcinoma cells in primary culture, but not normal cells, and the induction of urokinase-PA secretion from carcinoma cells. It was presumed that both effects were mediated via direct activation of protein kinase C, since TPA is known to increase urokinase-PA mRNA synthesis (Stoppelli *et al.*, 1986). Thus, diglycerides might act as endogenous mitogens in the development of human colon cancer, selecting only for pre-malignant and malignant cell growth. Marian *et al.*

(1990) demonstrated that the faecal diglyceride dimyristin released 17 times more urokinase from carcinoma cells than from normal colonocytes. This increase in the steady-state level of urokinase secretion was strongly dependent on the chain lengths of the fatty acid residues. Those with 14 and 16 carbon chains had the greatest activity. Thus, faecal diglycerides composed of oleic, myristic and palmitic acid residues induce two selective biological responses in colon tumour cells, namely mitogenesis and the secretion of urokinase-PA. One could propose, therefore, that mitogenesis might increase the adenoma and carcinoma cell numbers relative to normal cells and that the induction of the proteolytic enzyme urokinase would aid local tumour invasion within the bowel wall (Blasi *et al.*, 1987; Markus, 1988).

Extracellular matrix interactions

The interaction of tumour cells with the basement membrane is a critical step in the initiation of tumour invasion and subsequent metastasis (Liotta *et al.*, 1986; Terranova *et al.*, 1986; Wewer *et al.*, 1987). Normal epithelia synthesise, assemble and adhere to a well-defined basement membrane (Timpl and Dziadek, 1986), the loss of which is associated with the neoplastic proliferation of epithelial tumours. Thus moderately well-differentiated tumours in tissue section contain regions of intact basement membrane, whilst poorly differentiated tumours contain very few (Barsky *et al.*, 1983; Daneker *et al.*, 1987; Forster *et al.*, 1984; Kellokumpu *et al.*, 1985; Burtin *et al.*, 1982). The extent of the intact basement membrane in tissue section is therefore one of the criteria used to establish degree of differentiation. Generally, poorly differentiated colon adenocarcinomas are more aggressive and have a worse prognosis (Steinberg *et al.*, 1986; Klimpfinger *et al.*, 1987; Mentges, 1987).

Daneker *et al.* (1989) established a series of human colorectal carcinoma cell lines from tumour tissue and classified them according to several criteria related to differentiation. The cell lines were defined as either moderately well or poorly differentiated depending on the histology of the original tumour, the histology of the xenografts they formed in experimental animals, their *in vitro* morphology and their expression of carcinoembryonic antigen. In these *in vitro* studies (Daneker *et al.*, 1989) the poorly differentiated cell lines adhered to surfaces coated with laminin or Matrigel (reconstituted basement membrane) (Kleinman *et al.*, 1986) to a significantly greater extent than did the moderately well differentiated cell lines. Previous studies (Bryant *et al.*, 1986; Wewer *et al.*, 1987) had suggested that metastatic tumour cells express increased amounts of laminin receptor compared with non-invasive cells. In addition, the poorly differentiated cell lines exhibited considerable spreading on laminin and Matrigel after adherence that was not observed for the moderately well-differentiated cell lines. The adherence of the same cell lines on fibronectin did not correlate well with differentiation, although generally poorly differentiated cell lines adhered better than moderately differentiated cell lines. The use of specific peptide inhibitors of laminin and fibronectin binding showed that the interaction of the different cell lines with the extracellular matrix components was related to the degree of differentiation of the original tumour.

During normal tissue growth, epithelial cells appear to interact preferentially with laminin, whilst mesenchymal cells interact preferentially with fibronectin (Ekblom *et al.*, 1986; Terranova *et al.*, 1986). Invasive carcinoma cells, however, migrate through stromal elements which presumably requires considerable interaction with fibronectin. Therefore, one can postulate that the increased invasive and metastatic potential of poorly differentiated colon carcinoma cells is related to the enhanced ability of these cells to interact with basement membrane components. However, it is dangerous to extrapolate too much because the loss and reduced expression of two cell adhesion molecules, E-cadherin (Frixen *et al.*, 1991) and DCC (Fearon and Vogelstein, 1990), has recently been associated with progression to carcinoma status and loss of differentiation. In the case of E-cadherin reduced expression has also been related to increased invasiveness, and a carcinoma-derived epithelial cell line, but not a pre-malignant adenoma-derived cell line, was shown to secrete mature forms of the cysteine proteinases cathepsins B and L (Maciewicz *et al.*, 1989). The secretion of proteinases from cells has also been implicated in tumour invasion and metastasis (Woolley, 1984; Gal and Gottesman, 1986; Liotta, 1986; Denhardt *et al.*, 1987). Tumour invasion and metastasis are complex phenomena and it seems likely that all these factors are involved, in varying combinations, in the evolution of the invasive and metastatic phenotypes of certain adenocarcinomas.

Chemotherapeutic drug sensitivity of colon carcinomas in monolayer culture

Historically, colon carcinoma is one of the tumours most refractory to treatment by chemotherapy (Moertel, 1975) and drug resistance is even observed in previously untreated tumours. Therefore it is important to identify the factors influencing the resistance of these tumours. The 20 per cent response rate of colorectal tumours to 5-fluorouracil (5-FU), has not been improved by administering it in combination with cisplatin (Dy *et al.*, 1986) or methotrexate (Canobbio *et al.*, 1986). Schroy *et al.* (1988)

tested ten previously untreated colorectal carcinomas for their sensitivity in monolayer culture to the drugs mitomycin C, cisplatin, streptozotocin and 5-FU. Each drug induced colony lysis, in a dose-dependent manner, in responsive tumours. Drug-resistant cycling cells were identified by thymidine incorporation into colonies that were not lysed by the treatment. Consistent with the poor clinical response of colorectal tumours to chemotherapeutic drugs, each of the ten carcinomas tested exhibited inherent resistance to one or more of the drugs tested, within clinically achievable concentration ranges.

Tumour heterogeneity (Nowell, 1976), involving the expression of drug-resistant phenotypes, is thought to be a contributing factor in the refractory nature of these tumours. Ferguson and Cheng (1989) addressed directly the problem of inherent phenotypic instability with respect to drug resistance, using a cloned colorectal carcinoma cell line (HCT-clone A). Clone A was passaged in culture in the absence of drug selection. During this time the sensitivity to several drugs was examined and found to decrease 4-fold over a period of 30 weeks. Five randomly selected subclones never exposed to drugs displayed a range of sensitivities to vincristine (9-fold) and etoposide, but not to methotrexate. With time these sensitivities changed and further subclones were chosen from these lines exhibiting highest and lowest sensitivities for various drugs. Again a wide range of phenotypes was observed, with a 14-fold range of sensitivity for vincristine and a 3-fold range for doxorubicin. Cellular accumulation of vincristine and expression of the *mdr* p-glycoprotein, also varied significantly between subclonal lines. Therefore, not only do individual carcinomas differ in their intrinsic drug sensitivities, but individual tumours may be phenotypically unstable with respect to drug sensitivity.

The mechanisms of acquired drug-resistance include amplification of target genes and of the 170 kDa *mdr* p-glycoprotein, elevated levels of glutathione transferase and glutathione peroxidase, and progression-linked imbalances in the pathways of purine and pyrimidine metabolism (Weber, 1983; Kinsella and Haran, 1991). The importance of the pathways of pyrimidine synthesis in drug resistance is indicated in two studies on the effects of 5-fluoropyrimidines on colon carcinoma cell lines (Lonn and Lonn, 1988; Lonn *et al.*, 1989). Thymidine added after treatment with 5-fluoropyrimidine partly rescued cells and reduced the level of DNA fragmentation (Lonn and Lonn, 1988). Dipyridamole, on the other hand, which inhibits the uptake of nucleosides from the medium and therefore the availability of substrates for the salvage pathways, induced high levels of DNA lesions and a concomitant increase in cytotoxicity (Lonn *et al.*, 1989). Previously a defect in nucleoside transport in the HCT-8 colon carcinoma cell line had been shown to confer resistance to 5-fluoro-2′-deoxyuridine (Sobrero *et al.*, 1985*a*). However the same cell line could not be protected from methotrexate-induced toxicity by thymidine for the very reason that the nucleoside transport was impaired in these cells (Sobrero *et al.*, 1985*b*).

Evaluation of risk factors and genotoxicity using bacterial and mammalian cell systems

In vitro model systems allow the rapid testing of some of the hypotheses concerning the roles of certain agents in the aetiology of colorectal carcinoma.

Over the years a large body of evidence has accumulated to support the concept that bile acids and their secondary metabolites act as promoters of colon carcinogenesis (Nigro and Campbell, 1976). In general, populations consuming higher amounts of fat have higher levels of bile acids and a higher risk for colon cancer. As stated previously (Chapter 4), the primary bile acids are cholic and chenodeoxycholic acids and the secondary bile acids lithocholic and deoxycholic acids. Lithocholic acid has been shown to cause alterations in the proliferative activity of deep cryptal colonic cells in culture (Turjman *et al.*, 1982), as well as to increase the incorporation of labelled thymidine into mouse liver and biliary tract epithelium (Bagheri *et al.*, 1978). This is consistent with the *in vivo* evidence in rats that bile acids can induce a proliferative response following the damage they produce in the surface epithelium (Bull *et al.*, 1983). Certainly, lithocholic and deoxycholic acid were markedly cytotoxic in several *in vitro* studies (Kelsey and Pienta, 1981; Kaibara *et al.*, 1984; Gaull and Wright, 1987). Lithocholic acid was shown to induce DNA strand breaks in mouse L1210 cells (Kulkarni *et al.*, 1980). It has also been shown to be co-mutagenic in the *Salmonella* mammalian microsome mutagenicity test (Silverman and Andrews, 1977; Wilpart *et al.*, 1983), although as discussed previously (Chapter 3) the evidence regarding the genotoxicity of bile acids is essentially negative (Venitt *et al.*, 1987; Venitt, 1988). However, Cheah and Bernstein (1990), using a M13 DNA transfection assay, suggested that bile acids are DNA damaging and that the DNA damage can be reduced by the presence of cellulose. Their thesis was that cellulose might act by inducing polyesterification of the bile acids to inactive forms.

Support for the suggestion that secondary bile acids and their metabolic products might act in concert with carcinogens to promote neoplastic transformation in the colon comes from studies in cell culture transformation model systems. Kelsey and Pienta (1981) showed lithocholic and deoxycholic acid to be more toxic than their primary bile acid precursors and to transform Syrian hamster embryo cells in culture. In the same study cholesterol, the metabolic precursor of bile acids, was inactive. Kaibara *et al.* (1984) showed both primary and secondary bile acids to enhance MNNG-induced neoplastic transformation in the $C_3H10T1/2$ mouse transformation assay system. Using the same $C_3H10T1/2$ transformation assay system, Kawasumi *et al.* (1988) showed lithocholic acid to enhance 3-methylcholanthrene (MCA)-induced transformation when added either simultaneously with or following MCA treatment. This suggested that bile acids might not only act as promoting agents but also as co-carcinogens, and strongly supports a role for bile acids in colon carcinogenesis.

In vitro studies in colon cancer cell lines suggest that individual polyamines may have a selective role in the expression of key growth-related genes such as c-*myc* and c-*fos* (Celano *et al.*, 1989), which can be modulated by specific inhibitors such as difluoromethylornithine (DFMO). DFMO, as discussed in Chapter 4, has been shown to be a useful inhibitor of tumourigenesis *in vivo* in rat model systems.

Although the epidemiological data suggest that selenium might be protective against colorectal carcinoma (Clark, 1985), the *in vitro* data are conflicting. Unusually for an agent that is protective against cancer, selenium in the form of sodium selenite is clastogenic in rat (Newton and Lilly, 1986) and human lymphocytes (Khalil, 1989). It is also mutagenic and cytotoxic in the *Salmonella* test (Kramer and Ames, 1988). Sodium selenite was shown to inhibit radiogenic and chemically induced transformation in the mouse $C_3H10T1/2$ system by virtue of its ability to induce free-radical scavenging systems and peroxide breakdown (Borek *et al.*, 1986). The same compound was shown to have a biphasic effect on the growth of mammary epithelial cells in culture, stimulating cell growth at low concentrations and inhibiting it at high concentrations (Medina and Osborn, 1984). In fact sodium selenite was shown to induce reversible, non-lethal inhibition of growth at low doses, whilst prolonged exposure to higher doses (5 μmol/l) was cytotoxic (Morrison and Medina, 1988). It may be, therefore, that selenium inhibits carcinogenesis by virtue of its ability to inhibit the proliferation of responsive cells.

The identification of genotoxicity in faecal extracts using *in vitro* mutagenicity testing is well documented (Bruce *et al.*, 1977; reviewed by Venitt, 1988). The novel class of direct-acting mutagens identified by these tests were called faecapentaenes and were shown to be the products of bacterial metabolism in the human colon. However, it is generally accepted that there is no difference between cancer patients and controls in their faecal genotoxicity. Therefore the evidence for a role for faecapentaenes in the causation of colorectal carcinoma is at best circumstantial. However, Curren *et al.* (1987) showed faecapentaene-12 to increase unscheduled DNA synthesis in both rat hepatocytes and human fibroblasts and to induce the neoplastic transformation of BalbC/3T3 mouse cells. Hinzman *et al.* (1987) showed faecapentaene-12 to damage mammalian colon DNA.

References

Antecol, M. H. and Mukherjee, B. B. (1982) Effect of 12-*O*-tetradecanoylphorbol-13-acetate on fibroblasts from individuals genetically predisposed to cancer. *Cancer Res.*, **42**, 3870–9.

Armitage, N. C., Robins, R. A., Evans, D. F., *et al.* (1985) The influence of tumour cell DNA abnormalities on survival in colorectal cancer. *Br. J. Surg.*, **72**, 828–30.

Bagheri, S. A., Bolt, M. S., Boyer, J. D. and Palmer, R. H. (1978) Stimulation of thymidine incorporation in mouse liver and biliary tract epithelium by lithocholate and deoxycholate. *Gastroenterology*, **74**, 188–92.

Baker, S. J., Fearon, E. R., Nigro, J. M., *et al.* (1989) Chromosome 17p deletions and p53 mutations in colorectal carcinomas. *Science*, **244**, 217–21.

Barsky, S. H., Siegal, G. P., Jannotta, F. and Liotta, L. A. (1983) Loss of basement membrane components by invasive tumours but not by their benign counterparts. *Lab. Invest.*, **49**, 140–7.

Blasi, F., Vassalli, J.-D. and Dano, K. (1987) Urokinase-type plasminogen activator proenzyme, receptor and inhibitors. *J. Cell Biol.*, **104**, 801–4.

Bogenmann, E. and Jones, P. A. (1983) Role of plasminogen in matrix breakdown by neoplastic cells. *J. Natl. Cancer Inst.*, **71**, 1177–82.

Borek, C., Ong, A., Mason, H., *et al.* (1986) Selenium and vitamin E inhibit radiogenic and chemically induced transformation *in vitro* via a different mechanism. *Proc. Natl. Acad. Sci. USA*, **83**, 1490–4.

Bos, J. L., Fearon, E. R., Hamilton, S. R., *et al.* (1987) Prevalence of *ras* gene mutations in human colorectal cancers. *Nature*, **327**, 293–7.

Brattain, M. G., Markes, M. E., McCombs, J., *et al.* (1983) Characterisation of human colon carcinoma cell lines isolated from a single primary tumour. *Br. J. Cancer*, **47**, 373–81.

Bruce, W. R., Varghese, A. J., Wang, S. and Land, P. C. (1977) A mutagen in the faeces of normal humans. In: *Origins of Human Cancer*, book C. ed. H. H. Hiatt *et al.*, pp. 1641–6. Cold Spring Harbor, New York.

Bryant, G., Haberen, C., Rao, C. N. and Liotta, L. A. (1986) Butyrate-induced reduction of tumour cell laminin receptors. *Cancer Res.*, **46**, 807–11.

Bull, A. W., Marnett, L. J., Dawe, E. J. and Nigro, N. D. (1983) Stimulation of thymidine incorporation in the colon of rats treated intrarectally with bile acids and fats. *Carcinogenesis*, **4**, 207–10.

Burtin, P., Chavanel, G., Foidart, J. M. and Martin, E. (1982) Antigens of the basement membrane and peritumoral stroma in human colonic adenocarcinoma: an immunofluorescence study. *Int. J. Cancer*, **30**, 13–20.

Cajot, J.-F., Kruithof, E. K. O., Schleuning, W. D., *et al.* (1986) Plasminogen activators, plasminogen activator inhibitors and procoagulant analysed in twenty human tumour cell lines. *Int. J. Cancer*, **38**, 719–27.

Canobbio, L., Nobile, M. T., Ardizzoni, A., *et al.* (1986) Phase II study of sequential methotrexate and 5-FU combination in the treatment of advanced colorectal cancer. *Cancer Treat. Rep.*, **70**, 419–20.

Carrel, S., Sordat, B. and Merenda, C. (1976) Establishment of a cell line (Co-115) from a human colon carcinoma transplanted into mice. *Cancer Res.*, **36**, 3978–84.

Celano, P., Berchtold, C. M., Giardiello, F. M. and Casaro, R. A. (1989) Modulation of growth gene expression by selective alteration of polyamines in human colon carcinoma cells. *Biochem. Biophys. Res. Commun.*, **165**, 384–90.

Clark, L. C. (1985) The epidemiology of selenium and cancer. *Fed. Proc.*, **44**, 2584–9.

Corasanti, J. G., Celik, C., Cambiolo, S. M., *et al.* (1980) Plasminogen activator content of human colon tumours and normal mucosae: separation of enzymes and partial purification. *J. Natl. Cancer Inst.*, **65**, 345–51.

Couturier-Turpin, M. H., Louvei, A., Courturier, D., *et al.* (1988) Tubulovillous adenoma of the colon with hyperdiploidy, double minute chromosomes and inversion of chromosome 1. *Cancer Genet. Cytogenet.*, **32**, 253–62.

Curren, R. D., Putman, D. L., Yang, L. L., *et al.* (1987) Genotoxicity of faecapentaene-12 in bacterial and mammalian cell assay systems. *Carcinogenesis*, **8**, 349–52.

Daneker, G. W., Mercurio, A. M., Guerra, L., *et al.* (1987) Laminin expression in colorectal carcinomas varying in degree of differentiation. *Arch. Surg.*, **122**, 1470–4.

Daneker, G. W., Piazza, A., Steele, G. D. and Mercurio, A. M. (1989) Relationship between extracellular matrix interactions and degree of differentiation in human colon carcinoma cell lines. *Cancer Res.*, **49**, 681–6.

Danes, B. S. (1976) The Gardner syndrome: increased tetraploidy in cultured skin fibroblasts. *J. Med. Genet.*, **13**, 52–6.

Danes, B. S. (1981) Occurrence of *in vitro* tetraploidy in the heritable colon cancer syndromes. *Cancer*, **48**, 1596–601.

Danes, B. S. (1985) Long-term cultured colon epithelial cell lines from individuals with and without colon cancer genotypes. *J. Natl. Cancer Inst.*, **75**, 261–7.

Danes, B. S. and Alm, T. (1981) *In-vitro* evidence of genetic heterogeneity within the heritable colon cancer syndromes with polyposis coli. *Scand. J. Gastroenterol.*, **16**, 421–7.

Danes, B. S., Boyle, P. D., Traganos, F. and Melamed, M. R. (1986) A standardised assay to identify colon cancer genotypes by *in vitro* tetraploidy in human dermal fibroblasts. *Disease Markers*, **4**, 271–82.

Danes, B. S., De Angelis, P., Traganos, F. and Melamed, M. R. (1988) Tetraploidy in cultured dermal fibroblasts from patients with heritable colon cancer. *Disease Markers*, **6**, 151–61.

De Bruin, P. A. F., Griffoen, G., Verspaget, H. W., *et al.* (1987) Plasminogen activators and tumour development in the human colon: activity levels in normal mucosa, adenomatous polyps and adenocarcinomas. *Cancer Res.*, **47**, 4654–7.

Delattre, P., Olschwang, S., Law, D. J., *et al.* (1989) Multiple genetic alterations distinguish distal from proximal colorectal cancer. *Lancet*, **2**, 353–6.

Delhanty, J. D. A., Davis, M. B. and Wood, J. (1983) Chromosome instability in lymphocytes, fibroblasts and colon-epithelial-like cells from patients with FPC. *Cancer Genet. Cytogenet.*, **8**, 27–50.

Denhardt, D. T., Greenberg, A. H., Egan, S. E., *et al.* (1987) Cystein proteinase cathepsin L expression correlates closely with metastatic potential of H-*ras* transformed murine fibroblasts. *Oncogene*, **2**, 55–9.

Deschner, E. and Lipkin, M. (1975) Proliferative patterns in colonic mucosa in familial polyposis. *Cancer*, **35**, 413–18.

Dy, C., Gil, A., Algarra, S. M., *et al.* (1986) Combination chemotherapy of cisplatin and 5FU in advanced colorectal carcinoma. *Cancer Treat. Rep.*, **70**, 465–8.

Ekblom, P., Vestweber, D. and Kemler, R. (1986) Cell matrix interactions and cell adhesion during development. *Annu. Rev. Cell Biol.*, **2**, 27–47.

Eliyahu, D., Michalovitz, D., Eliyahu, S., *et al.* (1989) Wild-type p53 can inhibit oncogene-mediated focus formation. *Proc. Natl. Acad. Sci. USA*, **86**, 8763–7.

Emdin, S. O., Stenling, R. and Roos, G. (1987) Prognostic value of DNA content in colorectal carcinoma. *Cancer*, **60**, 1282–7.

Fearon, E. R. and Vogelstein, B. (1990) A genetic model for colorectal tumorigenesis. *Cell*, **61**, 759–67.

Fearon, E. R., Hamilton, S. R. and Vogelstein, B. (1987) Clonal analysis of human colorectal tumours. *Science*, **238**, 193–7.

Fearon, E. R., Cho, K. R., Nigro, J. M., *et al.* (1990) Identification of a chromosome 18q gene that is altered in colorectal cancers. *Science*, **247**, 49–56.

Ferguson, P. J. and Cheng, Y. C. (1989) Phenotypic instability of drug sensitivity in human colon carcinoma cell line. *Cancer Res.*, **49**, 1148–53.

Ferti, A. D., Panani, A. D. and Raptis, S. (1988) Cytogenetic study of rectosigmoidal adenocarcinomas. *Cancer Genet. Cytogenet.*, **34**, 101–9.

Finlay, C. A., Hinds, P. W. and Levine, A. J. (1989) The p53 protooncogene can act as a suppressor of transformation. *Cell*, **57**, 1083–93.

Forrester, K., Almoguera, C., Han, K., *et al.* (1987) Detection of a high incidence of K-*ras* oncogenes during human colon tumourigenesis. *Nature*, **327**, 298–303.

Forslund, G., Cedermark, B., Ohman, U., *et al.* (1984) The significance of DNA distribution pattern in rectal carcinoma: a preliminary study. *Dis. Colon Rectum*, **27**, 579–84.

Forster, S. J., Talbot, I. C. and Critchley, D. R. (1984) Laminin and fibronectin in rectal adenocarcinoma: relationship to tumour grade, stage and metastasis. *Br. J. Cancer*, **50**, 51–61.

Friedlander, M. L., Hedley, D. W. and Taylor, I. W. (1984) Clinical and biological significance of aneuploidy in human tumours. *J. Clin. Pathol.*, **37**, 961–97.

Friedman, E. (1981) Differential response of epithelial cell classes to phorbol ester tumour promoters and to deoxycholic acid. *Cancer Res.*, **41**, 4588–91.

Friedman, E., Gillin, S. and Lipkin, M. (1984*a*) 12-*O*-tetradecanoylphorbol-13-acetate stimulation of DNA synthesis in cultured preneoplastic familial polyposis colonic epithelial cells, but not in normal colonic epithelial cells. *Cancer Res.*, **44**, 4078–86.

Friedman, E., Urmacher, C. and Winawer, S. (1984*b*) A model for human colon carcinoma evolution based on the differential response of cultured preneoplastic, premalignant and malignant cells to 12-*O*-tetradecanoylphorbol-13-acetate. *Cancer Res.*, **44**, 1568–78.

Friedman, E., Isaksson, P., Rafter, J., *et al.* (1989) Fecal diglycerides as selective endogenous mitogens for premalignant and malignant human colonic epithelial cells. *Cancer Res.*, **49**, 544–8.

Frixen, U. H., Behrens, J., Sachs, M., *et al.* (1991) E-cadherin-mediated cell–cell adhesion prevents invasiveness in human carcinoma cells. *J. Cell. Biol.*, **113**, 173–85.

Gainer, H. St.C., Schor, S. and Kinsella, A. R. (1984) Susceptibility of skin fibroblasts from individuals genetically predisposed to cancer to transformation by the tumor promoter 12-*O*-tetradecanoylphorbol-13-acetate. *Int. J. Cancer*, **34**, 349–57.

Gal, S. and Gottesman, M. M. (1980) The major excreted protein of transformed fibroblasts is an activable acid-protease. *J. Biol. Chem.*, **261**, 1760–5.

Gardner, E. J., Rogers, S. W. and Woodward, S. (1982) Numerical and structural chromosome aberrations in cultured lymphocytes and cutaneous fibroblasts from patients with multiple adenomas of the colorectum. *Cancer*, **49**, 1413–19.

Gardner, E. J., Woodward, S. R. and Hughes, J. P. (1985) Evaluation of chromosome diagnosis for hereditary adenomatosis of the colorectum. *Cancer Genet. Cytogenet.*, **15**, 321–34.

Gaull, G. E. and Wright, C. E. (1987) Taurine conjugation of bile acids protects human cells in culture. *Adv. Exp. Med. Biol.*, **217**, 61–7.

Cheah, P. Y. and Bernstein, H. (1990) Colon cancer and dietary fibre: cellulose inhibits the DNA-damaging ability of bile acids. *Nutr. Cancer*, **13**, 15–17.

Goh, H. S. and Jass, J. R. (1986) DNA content and the adenoma–carcinoma sequence in the colorectum. *J. Clin. Pathol.*, **39**, 387–92.

Hamada, S., Namura, K., Itoh, R. and Fujita, S. (1987) Characteristics of colorectal epithelia and adenomas as revealed by DNA cytofluorometry. *Jpn. J. Cancer Res.*, **78**, 826–32.

Hastie, N. D., Dempster, M., Dunlop, M., *et al.* (1990) Telomere reduction in human colorectal carcinoma and with ageing. *Nature*, **346**, 866–8.

Heim, S. (1985) Spontaneous and mitomycin C induced structural chromosome aberrations in lymphocytes from patients with adenomatosis of the colon and rectum. *Hereditas*, **103**, 235–8.

Heim, S., Johansen, S. G., Kolnig, A.-M. and Strombeck, B. (1984) Increased levels of spontaneous and mutagen-induced chromosome aberrations in skin fibroblasts from patients with adenomatosis of the colon and rectum. *Cancer Genet. Cytogenet.*, **17**, 333–46.

Hiddemann, W., Schumann, J., Andreef, M., *et al.* (1984) Convention on nomenclature for DNA cytometry. *Cytometry*, **5**, 445–6.

Hinzman, M. J., Novotny, C., Ullah, A. and Shamsuddin, A. M. (1987) Faecal mutagen faecapentaene-12 damages mammalian colon epithelial DNA. *Carcinogenesis*, **8**, 1475–9.

Hori, T., Murata, M. and Utsunomiya, J. (1980) Chromosome aberrations induced by *N*-methyl-*N*′-nitro-*N*-nitrosoguanidine in cultured skin fibroblasts from patients with adenomatous coli. *Gann.*, **71**, 628–36.

Iwana, T., Utsunomiya, J. and Sasaki, J. (1977) Epithelial cell kinetics in the crypt of familial polyposis of the colon. *Jpn. J. Surg.*, **7**, 230–4.

Jenkyn, D. J., Whitehead, R. H., House, A. K. and Maley, M. A. L. (1987) A single chromosome defect, partial trisomy 1q, in a colon cancer cell line. *Cancer Genet. Cytogenet.*, **27**, 357–60.

Jones, D. J., Moore, M. and Schofield, P. F. (1988) Prognostic significance of DNA ploidy in colorectal cancer: a prospective flow cytometric study. *Br. J. Surg.*, **75**, 28–33.

Kaibara, N., Yurugi, E. and Koga, S. (1984) Promoting effect of bile acids on the chemical transformation of C_3H10T1/2 fibroblasts *in vitro*. *Cancer Res.*, **44**, 5482–5.

Kawasumi, H., Kaibara, N. and Koga, S. (1988) Carcinogenic activity of bile acids in the chemical transformation of C_3H10T1/2 fibroblasts *in vitro*. *Oncology*, **45**, 192–6.

Kellokumpu, I., Ekblom, P. and Scheinin, T. M. (1985) Malignant transformation in human colorectal mucosa as monitored by distribution of laminin a basement membrane glycoprotein. *Acta Pathol. Microbiol. Immunol. Scand.*, **93**, 285–91.

Kelsey, M. I. and Pienta, R. J. (1981) Transformation of hamster embryo cell by neutral sterols and bile acids. *Toxicol. Lett.*, **9**, 177–82.

Khalil, A. M. (1989) The induction of chromosome aberrations in human purified peripheral blood lymphocytes following *in vitro* exposure to selenium. *Mutat. Res.*, **224**, 503–6.

Kinsella, A. R. (1988) The study of multi-stage carcinogenesis in retinoblastoma and familial polyposis coli patient-derived skin fibroblast cell culture system. *Mutat. Res.*, **119**, 353–68.

Kinsella, A. R. and Gainer, H. St.C. (1984) *In vitro* studies of the possible mechanisms whereby tumour promoters mediate their responses. In: *Cellular Interactions of Environmental Tumour Promoters*, ed. H. Fujiki *et al.*, pp. 261–72. Japan Sci. Soc. Press/VNU Press, Utrecht.

Kinsella, A. R. and Haran, M. S. (1991) Decreasing sensitivity to cytotoxic agents parallels increasing tumourigenicity in human fibroblasts. *Cancer Res.*, **51**, 1855–9.

Kleinman, H. K., McGarvey, M. L., Hassell, J. R., *et al.* (1986) Basement membrane complexes with biological activity. *Biochemistry*, **25**, 312–18.

Klimpfinger, M., Beham, A. and Denk, H. (1987) Pathologic findings in colorectal cancers and discussion of their significance for tumour therapy according to stage. *Wien. Klin. Wochenschr.*, **99**, 488–93.

Kokal, W., Sheibani, K., Terz, J. and Harada, J. R. (1986) Tumour DNA content in the prognosis of colorectal carcinoma. *JAMA*, **255**, 3123–7.

Kopelovich, L. (1981) The use of a tumour promoter as a single parameter approach for the detection of individuals genetically predisposed to colorectal cancer. *Cancer Lett.*, **12**, 67–74.

Kopelovich, L. and Sirlin, S. (1980) Human skin fibroblasts from individuals genetically predisposed to cancer are sensitive to an SV-40-T antigen display and transformation. *Cancer*, **45**, 1108–11.

Kopelovich, L., Bias, N. E. and Helson, L. (1979) Tumour promoter alone induces malignant transformation of fibroblasts from humans genetically predisposed to cancer. *Nature*, **282**, 619–21.

Kopelovich, L., Lipkin, M., Blattner, W. A., *et al.* (1980) Organisation of actin-containing cables in cultured skin fibroblasts from individuals at high risk of colon cancer. *Int. J. Cancer*, **26**, 301–7.

Kopelovich, L., Drozdoff, V. and Zeitz, L. (1981) Transformation of human cell mutants by γ-irradiation. *Proc. Am. Assoc. Cancer Res.*, **21**, 192.

Kovacs, G. (1978) Abnormalities of chromosome 1 in human solid malignant tumours. *Int. J. Cancer*, **21**, 688–94.

Kramer, G. F. and Ames, B. N. (1988) Mechanisms of mutagenicity and toxicity of sodium selenite in *Salmonella typhimurium. Mutat. Res.*, **201**, 169–80.

Kulkarni, M. S., Heidepreim, P. M. and Yielding, K. L. (1980) Production by lithocholic acid of DNA strand breaks in L1210 cells. *Cancer Res.*, **40**, 2666–9.

Liebovitz, A., Stinson, J. C., McCombs, W. B., *et al.* (1976) Classification of human adenocarcinoma cell lines. *Cancer Res.*, **36**, 4562–9.

Liotta, L. A. (1986) Tumour invasion and metastasis: role of extracellular matrix. *Cancer Res.*, **46**, 1–7.

Liotta, L. A., Goldfarb, R. H., Brundage, R., *et al.* (1981) Effect of plasminogen activator (urokinase), plasmin and thrombin on glycoprotein and collagenous components of the basement membrane. *Cancer Res.*, **41**, 4629–36.

Liotta, L. A., Rao, C. N. and Weiner, V. M. (1986) Biochemical interactions of tumour cells with the basement membrane. *Annu. Rev. Biochem.*, **55**, 1037–55.

Lipkin, M. (1974) Phase 1 and Phase 2 proliferative lesions of colonic epithelial cells in diseases leading to colon cancer. *Cancer*, **34**, 878–88.

Lipkin, M., Blattner, W. E., Fraumeni, J. F., *et al.* (1983) Tritated thymidine labelling distribution as a marker for hereditary predisposition to colon cancer. *Cancer Res.*, **43**, 1899–904.

Lofberg, R., Tribukait, B., Ost, A., *et al.* (1957) Flow cytometric DNA analysis in longstanding ulcerative colitis: a method of prediction of dysplasia and carcinoma development. *Gut*, **28**, 1100–6.

Lonn, U. and Lonn, S. (1988) Increased levels of DNA lesions induced by leucovorin-5-fluoropyrimidine in human colon adenocarcinoma. *Cancer Res.*, **48**, 4153–7.

Lonn, U., Lonn, S., Nylen, U. and Winblad, G. (1989) 5-fluoropyrimidine-induced DNA damage in human colon adenocarcinoma and its augmentation by the nucleoside transport inhibitor dipyridamole. *Cancer Res.*, **49**, 1085–9.

Lothe, R. A., Gedde-Dahl, T., Lier, M. E., *et al.* (1987) Loss of one chromosome 13 during development of a polyposis tumour. *Cancer Genet. Cytogenet.*, **28**, 335–42.

Lukeis, R., Garson, O. M., Macrae, F. A., *et al.* (1987) Chromosome studies in inherited non-polyposis cancer syndrome. *Cancer Genet. Cytogenet.*, **27**, 111–24.

Maciewicz, R. A., Wardale, R. J., Etherington, D. J. and Paraskeva, C. (1989) Immunodetection of cathepsins B and L present in and secreted from human pre-malignant and malignant colorectal tumour cell lines. *Int. J. Cancer*, **43**, 478–86.

Marian, B., Harvey, S., Infante, D., *et al.* (1990) Urokinase secretion from human colon carcinomas induced by endogenous diglycerides. *Cancer Res.*, **50**, 2245–50.

Markus, G. (1988) The relevance of plasminogen activators to neoplastic growth. *Enzyme*, **40**, 158–72.

Medina, D. and Osborn, C. J. (1984) Selenium inhibition of DNA synthesis in mouse mammary epithelial cell line YN-4. *Cancer Res.*, **44**, 4361–5.

Mentges, B. (1987) Colon carcinoma: preoperative CEA, tumour differentiation and prognosis. *Dtsch. Med. Wochenschr.*, **112**, 1245–9.

Miller, R. W. and Todaro, G. J. (1969) Viral transformation of cells from persons at high risk of cancer. *Lancet*, **1**, 81–2.

Moertel, C. G. (1975) Clinical management of advanced gastrointestinal cancer. *Cancer*, **36**, 675–82.

Monpezat, J.-P., Delattre, O., Bernard, A., *et al.* (1988) Loss of alleles on chromosome 18 and on the short arm of 17 in polyploid colorectal tumours. *Int. J. Cancer*, **41**, 404–8.

Morrison, D. G. and Medina, D. (1988) Distinguishing features of cytotoxic and pharmacological effects of selenite in murine mammary epithelial cells *in vitro*. *Toxicol. Lett.*, **44**, 307–14.

Morson, B. C. (1974) The polyp–cancer sequence in the large bowel. *Proc. R. Soc. Med.*, **67**, 451–7.

Muleris, M., Salmon, R. J., Zafrant, B., *et al.* (1985) Consistent deficiencies of chromosome 18 and the short arm of chromosome 17 in eleven cases of human large bowel cancer: a possible recessive determinism. *Ann. Genet.*, **28**, 206–13.

Muleris, M., Salman, R. J., Dutrillaux, A. M., *et al.* (1987) Characteristic chromosomal imbalances in 18 near-diploid colorectal tumours. *Cancer Genet. Cytogenet.*, **29**, 289–301.

Muleris, M., Nordlinger, B. and Dutrillaux, B. (1989) Cytogenetic characterisation of a colon adenocarcinoma from a familial polyposis coli patient. *Cancer Genet. Cytogenet.*, **38**, 249–53.

Namba, M., Miyamoto, K., Hyodon, F., *et al.* (1983) Establishment and characterisation of a human colon carcinoma cell line (KMS-4) from a patient with hereditary adenomatosis of the colon and rectum. *Int. J. Cancer*, **32**, 697–702.

Newton, M. F. and Lilly, L. J. (1986) Tissue specific clastogenic effects of chromium and selenium salts *in vivo*. *Mutat. Res.*, **169**, 61–9.

Nigro, N. D. and Campbell, R. C. (1976) Bile acids and intestinal cancer. In: *The Bile Acids*, ed. P. P. Nair and D. Kitchevsky, pp. 155–68. Plenum Press, New York.

Nigro, J. M., Baker, S. J., Preisinger, A. C., *et al.* (1989) Mutations in p53 occur in diverse tumour types. *Nature*, **342**, 705–7.

Nowell, P. C. (1976) The clonal evolution of tumour cell populations. *Science*, **194**, 23–8.

Pareskeva, C., Buckle, B. G., Sheer, D. and Wigley, C. B. (1984) The isolation and characterisation of colorectal epithelial cell lines at different stages in malignant transformation from familial polyposis coli patients. *Int. J. Cancer*, **34**, 49–56.

Paraskeva, C., Finerty, S., Mountford, R. A. and Powell, S. C. (1989*a*) Specific cytogenetic abnormalities in two new human colorectal adenoma derived epithelial cell lines. *Cancer Res.*, **49**, 1282–6.

Paraskeva, C., Harvey, A., Finerty, S. and Powell, S. (1989*b*) Possible involvement of chromosome 1 in *in vitro* immortalisation: evidence from progression of a human adenoma derived cell line *in vitro*. *Int. J. Cancer*, **43**, 743–6.

Petersen, S. E. and Fiedrich, U. (1986) A comparison between flow cytometric ploidy investigation and chromosome analysis of 32 human colorectal tumours. *Cytometry*, **1**, 307–12.

Pfeffer, L. and Kopelovich, L. (1977) Differential genetic susceptibility of cultured human skin fibroblasts to transformation by Kirsten Murine Sarcoma Virus. *Cell*, **10**, 313–20.

Pfeffer, L., Lipkin, M., Stutman, O. and Kopelovich, L. (1976) Growth abnormalities of cultured skin fibroblasts derived from individuals with hereditary adenomatosis of the colon and rectum. *J. Cell Physiol.*, **89**, 29–38.

Ponder, B. A. J. (1988) Gene losses in human tumours. *Nature*, **335**, 400–2.

Quirke, P., Fozard, J. B. J., Dixon, M. F., *et al.* (1986) DNA aneuploidy in colorectal adenomas. *Br. J. Cancer*, **53**, 477–81.

Quirke, P., Dixon, M. F., Clayden, A. D., *et al.* (1987) Prognostic significance of DNA aneuploidy and cell proliferation in rectal adenocarcinomas. *J. Pathol.*, **151**, 285–91.

Rasheed, S. and Gardner, M. B. (1981) Growth properties and susceptibility to viral transformation of skin fibroblasts from individuals at high genetic risk of colorectal cancer. *J. Natl. Cancer Inst.*, **66**, 43–9.

Reichmann, A., Martin, P. and Levin, B. (1984) Chromosomes in large bowel tumours: a study of chromosome #1. *Cancer Genet. Cytogenet.*, **12**, 295–301.

Remvikos, Y., Muleris, M., Vielh, P., *et al.* (1988) DNA content and genetic evolution of human colorectal adenocarcinoma: a study by flow cytometry and cytogenetic analysis. *Int. J. Cancer*, **42**, 539–43.

Rhim, J. S., Huebner, R. J., Arenstein, P. and Kopelovich, L. (1980) Chemical transformation of ACR cells. *Int. J. Cancer*, **26**, 565–9.

Saadi, A. A., Palutke, M. and Krishna-Kumar, G. (1980) Evolution of chromosomal abnormalities in sequential cytogenetic studies of ataxia telangiectasia. *Hum. Genet.*, **55**, 23–9.

Sagar, R. (1989) Tumour suppressor genes: the puzzle and the promise. *Science*, **246**, 1406–12.

Sappino, A. P., Busso, N., Belin, D. and Vassalli, J. D. (1987) Increase of urokinase-type plasminogen activator gene expression in human lung and breast carcinomas. *Cancer Res.*, **47**, 4043–6.

Sasaki, M., Okamoto, M., Sato, C., *et al.* (1989) Loss of constitutional heterozygosity in colorectal tumours from patients with familial polyposis coli and those with non-polyposis colorectal carcinoma. *Cancer Res.*, **49**, 4402–6.

Schroeder, T. M. and German, J. (1974) Bloom's syndrome and Fanconi's anaemia. Demonstration of two distinctive patterns of chromosome disruption and rearrangement. *Hum. Genet.*, **25**, 299–306.

Schroeder, T. M. and Kurth, R. (1971) Spontaneous chromosomal breakage and high incidence of leukaemia in inherited disease. *Blood*, **37**, 96–112.

Schroy, P. C., Cohen, A., Winawer, S. J. and Friedman, E. A. (1988) New chemotherapeutic drug sensitivity assay for colon carcinomas in monolayer culture. *Cancer Res.*, **48**, 3236–44.

Schutte, B., Reynders, M. M. J., Wiggers, T., *et al.* (1987) Retrospective analysis of the prognostic significance of DNA content and proliferative activity in large bowel carcinoma. *Cancer Res.*, **47**, 5494–6.

Schwartz, D., Banner, B. F., Roseman, D. O. L. and Coon, J. S. (1986) Origin of multiple primary colon carcinomas. *Cancer*, **58**, 2082–8.

Sciallero, S., Bruno, S., Divinci, A., *et al.* (1988) Flow cytometric DNA ploidy in colorectal adenomas and family history of colorectal carcinoma. *Cancer*, **61**, 114–20.

Scott, N. A., Weiland, L. H., Dozois, R. R., Beart, R. W. and Lieber, M. M. (1987*a*) DNA aneuploidy in solitary colonic adenomas and the future risk of colorectal cancer. *Dis. Colon Rectum*, **31**, 423–6.

Scott, N. A., Grande, J. P., Weiland, L. H., *et al.* (1987*b*) Flow cytometric DNA patterns from colorectal cancers: how reproducible are they? *Mayo Clin. Proc.*, **62**, 331–7.

Shabtai, F., Sternberg, A., Klar, D., *et al.* (1986) Familial fragile 8q22 involved as a cancer break point in cells of a large bowel tumour. *Cancer Genet. Cytogenet.*, **31**, 113–18.

Silverman, S. J. and Andrews, A. W. (1977) Bile acids: co-mutagenic activity in the *Salmonella* mammalian microsome mutagenicity test. *J. Natl. Cancer Inst.*, **59**, 1557–9.

Sobrero, A. F., Moir, R. D., Bertino, J. R. and Handschumacher, R. E. (1985*a*) Defective facilitated diffusion of nucleotides, a primary mechanism of resistance to 5-fluoro-2′-deoxyuridine in HCT-8 tumour carcinoma line. *Cancer Res.*, **45**, 3155–60.

Sobrero, A., Handschumacher, R. E. and Bertino, J. R. (1985*b*) Highly selective drug combinations for human colon cancer cells resistant in vitro to 5-fluoro-2′-deoxyuridine. *Cancer Res.*, **45**, 3161–3.

Solomon, E., Voss, R., Hall, V., *et al.* (1987) Chromosome 5 allele loss in human colorectal carcinomas. *Nature*, **328**, 616–19.

Steinberg, S. M., Barwich, K. W. and Stablein, D. M. (1980) Importance of tumour pathology and morphology in patients with surgically resected colon cancer: findings from the Gastrointestinal Tumour Study Group. *Cancer*, **58**, 1340–5.

Stoppelli, P., Verde, P., Grimaldi, G., *et al.* (1986) Increase in urokinase plasminogen activator mRNA synthesis in human carcinoma cells in a primary effect of the potent tumour promoter phorbol myristate acetate. *J. Cell Biol.*, **102**, 1231–5.

Svendsen L. B., Lauristen, K. B., Bulow, S. and Danes, B. S. (1985) Increased *in vitro* tetraploidy: a possible biomarker for non-heritable colorectal cancer. *Scand. J. Gastroenterol.*, **20**, 1110–14.

Svendsen, L. B., Bulow, S., Sondergaard, J. O., *et al.* (1987*a*) *In vitro* tetraploidy in patients with non-hereditary colorectal adenoma and carcinoma. *Scand. J. Gastroenterol.*, **22**, 106–10.

Svendsen, L. B., Sondergaard, J. O., Hegnhoj, L., *et al.* (1987*b*) *In vitro* tetraploidy in patients with ulcerative colitis. *Scand. J. Gastroenterol.*, **22**, 601–5.

Svendsen, L. B., Larsen, J. K. and Christensen, I. J. (1989) Human skin fibroblast *in vitro* tetraploidy: flow cytometric DNA assay used to confirm metaphase assay in patients with various colonic diseases. *Cancer Genet. Cytogenet.*, **39**, 243–51.

Suzumiya, J., Hasui, Y., Kohga, S., *et al.* (1988) Comparative study of plasminogen activator antigens in colonic carcinomas and adenomas. *Int. J. Cancer*, **42**, 627–32.

Terranova, V. P., Hujanen, E. S. and Martin, G. R. (1986) Basement membrane and the invasive activity of metastatic tumour cells. *J. Natl. Cancer Inst.*, **77**, 311–16.

Timpl, R. and Dziadek, M. (1986) Structure, development and molecular pathology of basement membranes. *Int. Rev. Exp. Pathol.*, **29**, 1–112.

Todaro, G. J. (1968) Variable susceptibility of human cell strains to SV40 transformation. *Natl. Cancer Inst. Monogr.*, **29**, 271–5.

Todaro, G. J., Green, H. and Swift, M. R. (1966) Susceptibility of human diploid fibroblast strains to transformation by SV40. *Science*, **153**, 1252–4.

Turjman, N., Jacob, C., Bhagaran, M. and Wityk, N. (1982) Effect of lithocholic acid on the incorporation of thymidine into DNA of proliferating rat colon epithelial cells. *Fed. Proc.*, **41**, 881–5.

Van den Ingh, H. F., Griffioen, G. and Cornelisse, C. J. (1985) Flow cytometry detection of aneuploidy in colorectal adenomas. *Cancer Res.*, **45**, 3392–7.

Venitt, S. (1988) Mutagens in human faeces and cancer of the large bowel. In: *Role of Gut Flora in Toxicity and Cancer*, pp. 399–460. Academic Press, New York.

Venitt, S., Bosworth, D. and Easton, D. F. (1987) Lack of mutagenic activity of bile acids in bacterial fluctuation tests. *Mutat. Res.*, **190**, 191–6.

Vogelstein, B., Fearon, E. R., Hamilton, S. R., *et al.* (1988) Genetic alterations during colorectal tumour development. *New Engl. J. Med.*, **319**, 525–32.

Weber, G. (1983) Biochemical strategy of cancer cells and design of chemotherapy. G. H. A. Clowes Memorial Lecture. *Cancer Res.*, **43**, 3466–92.

Wewer, U. M., Taraboletti, G., Sobel, M. E., *et al.* (1987) Role of laminin receptor in tumour cell migration. *Cancer Res.*, **47**, 5691–8.

Whitehead, F., Jarvis, L. R., Skinner, J. M. and Whitehead, R. (1985) Ploidy studies in adenomatous polyps of the colon. *J. Clin. Pathol.*, **38**, 1261–4.

Wildrick, D. M. and Boman, B. M. (1988) Chromosome 5 allele loss at the glucocorticoid receptor locus in human colorectal carcinomas. *Biochem. Biophys. Res. Commun.*, **150**, 591–8.

Williams, A. C., Harper, S. and Paraskeva, C. (1990) Neoplastic transformation of a human colonic epithelial cell line: *in vitro* evidence for the adenoma–carcinoma sequence. *Cancer Res.*, **50**, 4724–30.

Wilpart, M., Mainguet, P., Maskens, A. and Roberfroid, M. (1983) Mutagenicity of 1,2-dimethylhydrazine towards *Salmonella typhimurium:* co-mutagenic effect of secondary bile acids. *Carcinogenesis*, **4**, 45–8.

Wilson, E. L., Becker, M. L. B., Hoal, E. G. and Dowdle, E. B. (1980) Molecular species of plasminogen activators secreted by normal and neoplastic human cells. *Cancer Res.*, **40**, 933–8.

Wolley, R. C., Schreiber, K., Koss, L. G., *et al.* (1982) DNA distribution in human colon carcinomas and its relationship to clinical behaviour. *J. Natl. Cancer Inst.*, **69**, 15–22.

Wolman, S. (1985) Chromosome markers in the study of colon cancer. *Dig. Dis. Sci.*, **30**, 1345–405.

Woolley, D. E. (1984) Collagenolytic mechanisms in tumour cell invasion. *Cancer Metast. Rev.*, **3**, 361–72.

6

Oncogenes and suppressor genes

DNAs from a variety of human tumours and human tumour cell lines have been shown to transform mouse NIH3T3 cells, leading to the identification of cellular transforming genes or oncogenes (Bishop, 1983; Cooper and Lane, 1984; Shih, 1984). The cellular transforming genes most frequently identified in this manner are three cellular oncogenes of the *ras* gene family: c-Ha-*ras*, c-Ki-*ras* and N-*ras*. Such studies also indicated that different members of the *ras* gene family were activated in different tumours of diverse origin, whilst the same *ras* gene was commonly, although not exclusively, associated with tumours of the same histological type.

Ras genes code for GTP binding proteins of molecular weight 21 kDa (p21) (Gibbs *et al.*, 1984; McGrath *et al.*, 1984; Sweet *et al.*, 1984) located on the inner surface of the plasma membrane, and are probably involved in the transduction of membrane-associated stimuli for cell proliferation (Bishop, 1983; Kamata and Feramisco, 1984). The activation of *ras* proto-oncogenes to oncogenes in human tumours is commonly due to point mutations at positions 12, 13 or 61 of the coding sequences. Such *ras* gene mutations result in diminished GTP hydrolysis by the *ras* protein, which in this form serves as a stimulus for malignant transformation. Recent studies have demonstrated Ki-*ras* mutations in an ever-increasing proportion of colorectal carcinomas (Bos *et al.*, 1987; Forrester *et al.*, 1987; Burmer and Loeb, 1989; Salhab *et al.*, 1989), although an activated Ha-*ras* gene with a mutation at codon 12 was identified in three colon carcinoma cell lines from the same patient (Greenhalgh and Kinsella, 1985) and an activated N-*ras* gene with a codon 13 mutation was identified in a colon carcinoma cell line (Cunningham and Weinberg, 1984) and a carcinoma of the rectum (Nitta *et al.*, 1987). Moreover, the coexistence of mutated Ki-

ras and N-*ras* genes has been reported in a colon carcinoma and a pre-invasive villous adenoma (Forrester *et al.*, 1987).

Although the majority of oncogene studies in colorectal carcinoma concern the *ras* gene family, other oncogenes have been studied and identified as being interesting in relation to the development of the disease. In particular attempts have been made to try to correlate levels of c-*myc* oncogene expression with the development of the disease. Allelic deletion of c-*myb* has also been reported and the human oncogene *trk* identified in a colon carcinoma (Mitra *et al.*, 1987); the *hst* gene has been identified in three stomach cancers and one colon cancer (Koda *et al.*, 1987).

Evolution of our understanding of *ras* oncogene involvement in colorectal carcinoma

During the first half of the 1980s, *ras* transforming genes were identified in approximately 15 per cent of all human solid tumours including colon carcinomas, using the NIH3T3 transformation assay system. The transforming genes identified in colorectal tumours and tumour cell lines using the NIH3T3 assay are detailed in Table 6.1; except for two instances they are members of the *ras* oncogene family.

Once the transforming genes predominantly involved in colorectal carcinoma had been identified as *ras* genes, the DNAs from the tumours and tumour cell lines could be analysed with specific restriction endonucleases for restriction fragment length polymorphisms (RFLPs), consistent with a specific mutation. There is strong evidence for the mechanism of *ras* gene activation being a mutation in the DNA coding sequence leading to an amino acid substitution at position 12, 13 or 61 in the *ras* gene product. For example in the case of the human Ha-*ras* gene, any mutation (e.g. G→T) in the sequence C<u>CGG</u> for codon 12, leads to a loss of the restriction site for *Msp*1 and *Hpa*11, facilitating the identification of a point mutation at this position. The normal sequence on digestion with *Msp*1 and *Hpa*11 produces a 355 base pair (bp) band and a 57 bp band, whilst the mutated form produces a 412 bp band on an agarose gel (Feinberg *et al.*, 1983; Greenhalgh and Kinsella, 1985).

In addition, the DNAs and RNAs from a wide variety of biopsy samples were analysed directly for amplification and elevated expression of the *ras* oncogene, which could be correlated with progression through the adenoma–carcinoma sequence, conventional Dukes' staging, differentiation state and aggressiveness of the disease. Spandidos and Kerr (1984) studied the expression of members of the *ras* oncogene family in premalignant polyps, malignant tumours and, where possible, the corre-

Table 6.1. *Transforming genes detected in colorectal tumours and tumour cell lines by NIH3T3 transfection*

DNA: tumour or cell line	Origin	Gene activated	Reference
CC20	Colon carcinoma cell line	Ha-*ras*	Greenhalgh and Kinsella (1985)
CC21	Colon carcinoma cell line	Ha-*ras*	
CC22	Colon carcinoma cell line	Ha-*ras*	
SKCO-1	Colon carcinoma cell line	Ki-*ras*	Perucho *et al.* (1981)
SW480	Colon carcinoma cell line	Ki-*ras*	Murray *et al.* (1981)
A2233	Colon carcinoma cell line	Ki-*ras*	Pulciani *et al.* (1982)
Duke 216	Colon carcinoma	Ki-*ras*	McCoy (1983)
CT1	Colon carcinoma	Ki-*ras*	Koda *et al.* (1987)
CT8	Colon carcinoma	Ki-*ras*	Koda *et al.* (1987)
Biopsy	Adenocarcinoma	N-*ras*	Murray *et al.* (1983)
7060	Rectal carcinoma metastasis	N-*ras*	Yuasa *et al.* (1986)
Biopsy	Rectal carcinoma	N-*ras*	Nitta *et al.* (1987)
CT9	Colon carcinoma	N-*ras*	Koda *et al.* (1987)
CT11	Colon carcinoma	N-*ras*	Koda *et al.* (1987)
CT14	Colon carcinoma	*HST*	Koda *et al.* (1987)
106-63	Colon carcinoma	*trk*	Martin-Zanca *et al.* (1986)

sponding normal mucosa (Table 6.2), using RNA spot hybridisation analysis. Quantification of the intensities of the autoradiographic spots was carried out by densitometric scanning. As can be seen (Table 6.2), transcripts from both Ki-*ras* and Ha-*ras* oncogenes could be detected in most malignant and pre-malignant tissue RNAs, but were barely detectable in normal tissue RNAs. The human *sis* oncogene, used as a control, was expressed at very consistent levels in all types of colonic tissues examined. Spandidos and Kerr (1984) concluded that the fact that Ki-*ras* and Ha-*ras* transcripts were elevated in both pre-malignant and malignant lesions when compared with the levels in the normal mucosa, showed that the increased expression of the *ras* genes was associated with the transformed state of the cells. However, as only a very few pre-malignant polyps or adenomas progress to malignancy, elevated *ras* gene expression alone can not be sufficient for transformation.

In the same year, Thor *et al.* (1984) suggested an alternative approach to determining whether or not a correlation existed between enhanced *ras* gene expression and progression to malignancy by using immunological methods directed against the p21 protein product. Using the monoclonal antibody RAP (*ras* peptide)-1, directed against a synthetic peptide com-

Table 6.2. *Expression of human c-Ki-*ras *and c-Ha-*ras *oncogenes in solid tumours, normal tissue and reference cell lines studied by RNA spot hybridisation analysis (Spandidos and Kerr, 1984)*

Patient		Normal[a]		Pre-malignant		Malignant	
No.	Origin	Ki-*ras*	Ha-*ras*	Ki-*ras*	Ha-*ras*	Ki-*ras*	Ha-*ras*
1	Colon	1.0	0.3	19[b]	31	6.3	4.5
2	Colon	2.0	3.5	20	8.0	3.5	14.0
3	Colon	2.0	2.3	9.5	9.1	19.0	9.0
4	Colon	1.7	1.0	—	—	7.0	7.6
5	Colon	2.3	1.0	—	—	3.5	1.5
6	Colon	1.0	1.0	—	—	6.5	1.5
7	Colon	1.0	1.3	—	—	7.0	1.5
8	Colon	4.1	1.5	2.2	8.0	—	—
9	Colon	—	—	—	—	5.0	1.5
10	Colon	—	—	—	—	4.4	1.5
11	Colon	—	—	—	—	6.5	11.0
12	Colon	—	—	—	—	1.9	14.0
13	Breast	—	—	—	—	3.0	6.3
CHB	Colon cell line	—	—	—	—	6.5	2.0
HL60	Promyelocytic	—	—	—	—	13.0	1.5
K562	Erythroleukaemic	—	—	—	—	8.0	1.5

Notes: [a]The figures represent arbitrary units assigned to the concentrations of HiHi3 (v-Ki-*ras*) or v-Ha-*ras* specific RNAs following scanning of autoradiographs.
[b]Patients 1 and 2, predominantly tubular polyps; patient 3, metaplastic polyp; and patient 8, tubulo-villous polyp.

prising amino acids 10–17 of human mutated *ras* p21 (Horan-Hand *et al.*, 1984), they investigated 47 colon carcinomas, 38 benign colonic lesions, including inflammatory and dysplastic lesions, and 18 specimens of normal colon from non-cancer patients for the presence of the p21 *ras* gene product in formalin-fixed sections. Of the 47 carcinomas examined, only 23 contained more than 20 per cent of cells staining for p21 (Fig. 6.1), whilst in the case of the 38 benign lesions 36 contained less than 5 per cent of cells staining for p21 (Fig. 6.1). Of the two remaining benign lesions, one was a tubulo-villous adenoma and the other was from a patient with diverticulitis. Neither showed more than 10 per cent of cells staining. The 18 normal colon samples showed essentially no staining (Fig. 6.1).

These differences in *ras* p21 expression in colon carcinomas when compared with normal colonic mucosa and benign colonic lesions, suggested that *ras* p21 expression might be correlated with depth of carcinoma and therefore was probably a relatively late event in colon carcinogenesis. However, although these data seemed very exciting, it had to be remembered that such antibodies had limitations. First, they did not distinguish between the normal and the mutated p21 molecules, and secondly they were only group-specific for human *ras* in that they identified a group of determinants shared by all *ras* genes and therefore did not distinguish between Ha-*ras*, Ki-*ras* or N-*ras*. Kerr *et al.* (1985), using the Y13-259 anti-p21 antibody (Furth *et al.*, 1982) on acetone-fixed frozen sections, showed p21 to be present in all epithelial populations of both pre-malignant and malignant colonic tumours. There was relatively weak, but apparently uniform staining of the epithelial cells of both normal adult and fetal colorectal crypts. A similar pattern was seen in

Fig. 6.1. Reactivity of RAP-1 with various colonic disease states on formalin-fixed sections. RAP-1 was reacted with adenocarcinomas (*a*, open circles), diverticulitis (*b*, filled circles), tubular adenomas (*b*, open squares), tubulo-villous adenomas (*b*, triangles), ulcerative colitis (*b*, crosses), hamartomatous polyps (*b*, filled squares) and normal colon (*c*, crosses) (after Thor *et al.*, 1984).

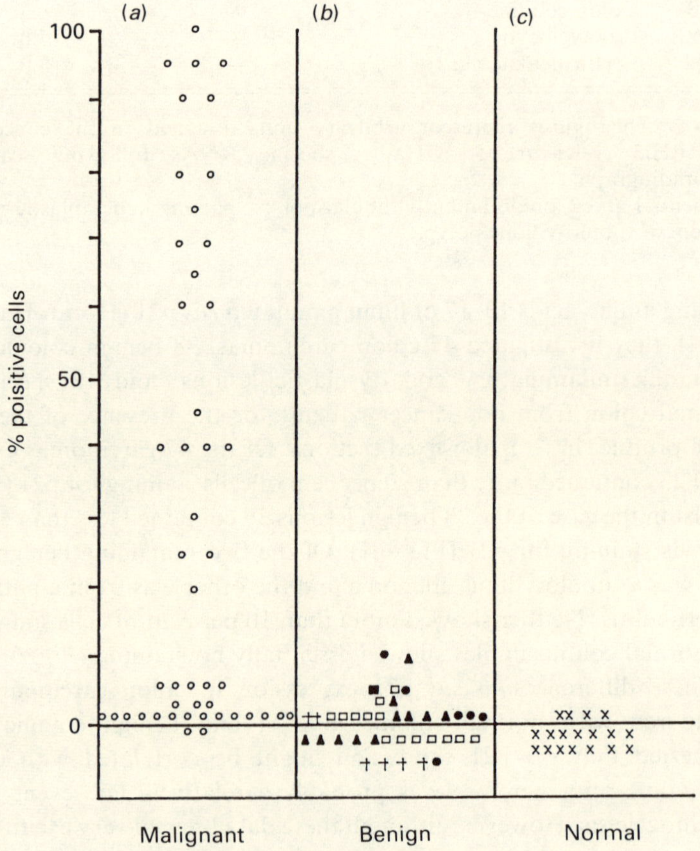

Table 6.3. *Staining intensity of colonic tissues for Y13-259 (Williams* et al., *1985)*

Tissue	No. of cases with staining intensity: ±	+	++
Carcinoma	15	4	2
Adenoma	0	1	5
Normal adjacent to carcinoma	7	9	0
Normal adjacent to adenoma	2	4	0
Normal non-neoplastic	4	3	0

Note: Adenomas show a significantly greater intensity of staining compared with carcinomas ($p<0.01$) and all normals ($p<0.002$) (four-fold table test). Carcinomas show no significant difference in staining intensity from normal mucosa.

adenomas and carcinomas, but the staining did appear to be more intense and less confined to the membrane than in normal tissues. However, Williams *et al.* (1985), using the same Y13-259 antibody, again on acetone-fixed frozen sections, showed that human colonic adenocarcinomas in general show a similar staining intensity to normal colonic mucosa, but that adenomas showed a consistently higher p21 expression as determined by staining intensity (Table 6.3).

Clearly, these data were different from those of Thor *et al.* (1984), suggesting that the two antibodies had different specificities – which was in fact confirmed by Robinson *et al.* (1986). This in turn throws some doubt on the more recent studies of Michelassi *et al.* (1987, 1988) using the RAP-5 antibody. However, the data of Williams *et al.* (1985) were consistent with the elevated *ras* transcripts reported by Spandidos and Kerr (1984) in adenomas and suggested that elevated *ras* gene expression may be important in the development of adenomas, but was less important as the tumour became more malignant and therefore more autonomous. Further confirmation of the importance of elevated *ras* gene expression in the early stages of colon tumour progression came from the studies of Gallick *et al.* (1985) using immunoblotting and the Y13-259 antibody. Of the 17 carcinomas analysed in this study (Table 6.4), nine had elevated levels of *ras*, seven had levels of *ras* equivalent to normal and one tumour had a lower level. Significantly, 4 of the 5 Dukes' D tumours (Astler Coller classification, Table 6.4) did not have elevated levels of *ras*.

Extension of these studies to colon metastases (Table 6.5) again confirmed that p21 levels were reduced compared with levels in normal tissues. The decreased levels of *ras* expression in tumours and metastases

Table 6.4. *Selected properties of primary colon tumours (Gallick* et al., *1985)*

Patient no.	Age	Sex	Dukes' stage[a]	p21 ratio tumour/adjacent normal[b]
1	50	M	C_2	>10
2	80	F	C_2	>10
3	52	F	B_2	>10
4	59	F	B_2	4.1
5	59	F	B_2	3.8
6	53	M	D	3.4
7	74	M	B_2	3.0
8	80	F	B_2	3.0
9	63	M	B_2	3.0
10	42	F	B_1	1.3
11	57	M	D	1.3
12	66	M	B_1	0.9
13	63	M	C_2	1.2
14	73	M	D	1.2
15	73	M	D	1.6
16	65	F	D	0.8
17	48	M	C_2	0.2

Notes: [a]The Astler Coller modification of the Dukes' system is used to classify colon tumours.
[b]p21 levels in tissue were determined by densitometry.

Table 6.5. *Selected properties of metastatic tumours from colon (Gallick* et al., *1985)*

Patient no.	Age	Sex	Site of metastasis[a]	p21 ratio tumour/normal colon[b]
1	72	M	Liver	<0.1
2	55	M	Liver	0.6
3	58	F	Liver	<0.1
4	61	M	Liver	<0.1
5	56	M	Lung	0.6
6	29	M	Lung	0.1
7	73	M	Lung	<0.1
8	50	F	Lung	<0.1
9	49	M	Omentum	0.5

Notes: [a]Pathology slides of primary and metastatic tumours were compared to determine that metastases were of colonic origin.
[b]Relative levels of p21 in tissue were determined by densitometry.

Table 6.6. *Classification of patients and tumours analysed for* ras *mutations (Bos* et al., *1987)*

Specimen	Dukes' stage	Location of tumour	*ras* mutations	Amino acid at mutated codon
s-7[a]	C	Recto-sigmoid	K12	Asp
S-15	C	Sigmoid	—	
S-16	A	Descending	K12	Asp
S-20	C	Ascending	—	
S-22[a]	C	Sigmoid	K12	Ser
S-27	A	Sigmoid	K12	Asp
S-32	A	Sigmoid	—	
S-42	B	Caecum	—	
S-43	C	Sigmoid	—	
S-45	A	Rectum	—	
S-46	B	Ascending	—	
S-89	B	Ascending	—	
S-92	B	Transverse	—	
S-93	C	Ascending	—	
S-94	A	Sigmoid	—	
S-95	C	Transverse	—	
S-96	A	Recto-sigmoid	—	
S-97	B	Sigmoid	K12	Asp
S-98	C	Caecum	N12	Cys
S-99	C	Caecum	—	
S-100[a]	C	Rectum	K12	Val
S-101[a]	B	Descending	K12	Val
S-102[a]	C	Sigmoid	K12	Asp
S-103	C	Ascending	—	
S-104	B	Ascending	—	
S-105[a]	C	Rectum	K61	His
S-106	C	Transverse	K12	Cys

Note: [a]Denotes tumours where comparison made with adenomas.

could be explained on the basis that tumour progression leads to increasing autonomy of the cell population and that concomitant with this lack of response to normal growth regulatory signals is the production of tumour growth factors. Production of tumour growth factors may alter *ras* gene expression or the expression of other oncogenes may alter *ras* gene expression.

However, although the work of Gallick *et al.* (1985) reinforced the evidence that there were changes in the levels of *ras* gene expression during tumour progression in colorectal cancer, the results rather surprisingly suggested that *ras* gene products with altered electrophoretic mobilities, consistent with mutational activation, were uncommon in the colon tumours analysed. Therefore, it was not until the work of Bos *et al.* (1987), in which small areas of the *ras* gene known to be 'hotspots' for mutation were amplified up from very small amounts of DNA isolated from very specific areas of paraffin sections, that any real clue to the frequency of *ras* mutations in colorectal malignancy could be assessed. Eleven out of 27 carcinomas analysed had a *ras* mutation, nine of Ki-*ras* 12, one of Ki-*ras* 61 and one of N-*ras* 12 (Table 6.6). Closer analysis of the data shows that not only are *ras* mutations found in advanced Dukes' B and C tumours, but also in two Dukes' A tumours at a relatively early stage in development before progression through the muscularis propria. Also, analysis of the six tumours asterisked in Table 6.6 which contained regions of both adenoma and carcinoma, showed five out of the six to have a mutation in both regions. As there is clear evidence that most colorectal tumours arise from pre-existing adenomas, these data suggest that *ras* gene alterations precede the development of malignancy. However, in one of the tumours (S7), a *ras* gene mutation was present only in the carcinoma and not in the adenoma suggesting, that the *ras* gene mutation also has a role to play in conversion to malignancy. These studies suggested two possible hypotheses for the role of *ras* genes in colorectal tumour progression: either mutations in *ras* genes may occur frequently in adenomas but only a small fraction of those adenomas with a mutation progress to malignancy, or *ras* mutations may occur infrequently in adenomas but those adenomas with *ras* mutations have a high probability of progression to the malignant state.

Forrester *et al.* (1987), using RNAse mismatch analysis of 66 primary human colon tumours, confirmed Ki-*ras* 12 mutations in 40 per cent. No apparent correlation was found between the presence of activated oncogenes and the degree of invasiveness of the tumour, but evidence for *ras* mutational activation in pre-malignant tumours was obtained. A high frequency of *ras* mutations was found in pre-malignant villous adenomas and in carcinomas originating from villous adenomas. The simultaneous presence of Ki-*ras* and N-*ras* oncogenes was demonstrated in an adenocarcinoma and a pre-invasive villous adenoma. These studies also suggested that mutations at the first position of codon 12 were present in the less invasive tumours whilst mutations present at the second position of codon 12 were commoner in more invasive tumours.

In the Manchester study (Salhab *et al.*, 1989) nine of the 31 colorectal carcinomas examined exhibited Ki-*ras* 12 mutations, nine had Ha-*ras* gene amplification alone, nine had Ki-*ras* gene amplification alone or in combination with a Ki-*ras* 12 mutation, and two exhibited both Ha-*ras* and Ki-*ras* gene amplification (Table 6.7). There was no correlation with Dukes' classification, grade or previous family history. Similarly there was

Table 6.7. ras *gene abnormalities in colorectal carcinomas (Salhab* et al., *1989)*

Sex	Age	Dukes' stage	Grade[a]	Ploidy[b]	History[c]
Ki-ras *mutation at codon 12*					
F	64	B	W	D	—
M	63	B	M	A	FH
F	76	B	M	A	—
Ki-ras *amplification*					
M	75	B	M	D	FH
M	50	C	M	D	FH[d]
F	45	C	M	D	—
Ki-ras *amplifications and codon 12 mutation*					
F	86	C	W	A	—[d]
M	62	B	W	D	FH
M	69	B	M	A	PH
M	90	B	M	A	PH
M	77	C	M	A	FH
M	66	C	M	D	—
Ha-ras *amplification*					
M	60	A	M	D	—
M	50	C	M	D	FH[d]
F	73	B	W	D	PH
F	80	B	M	D	PH
F	86	C	W	A	—[d]
F	81	B	P	A	PH
F	64	C	W	A	—
F	80	A	P	A	—
M	78	B	M	A	—
F	63	C	W	A	—
M	60	C	M	A	—
Normal ras *genes*					
M	48	B	W	A	—
M	49	B	M	D	—
M	72	C	M	A	—
M	62	B	M	A	—
F	49	B	M	D	—
F	45	C	M	A	—
F	35	B	M	A	FAP
M	50	C	M	A	—
M	33	B	M	D	FH
F	42	B	M	—	FH

Notes: [a]Grade of differentiation: M, moderate; P, poor; W, well.
[b]A, aneuploid; D, diploid.
[c]FH, family history of colorectal neoplasia; PH, previous history of colorectal neoplasia; FAP, familial adenomatous polyposis.
[d]Ki-*ras* and Ha-*ras* abnormalities in same tumour.

no correlation with ploidy, there being an equal distribution of aneuploid and diploid tumours with gene mutations and amplification. This again suggests that *ras* gene changes may be early events. Immunohistochemical staining of the same tumours using the Y13-259 anti-p21 antibody (Furth *et al.*, 1982) showed normal mucosa to exhibit membrane-associated staining which was common throughout the crypt. Three benign polyps were also stained and revealed membrane staining, whilst in the carcinomas the staining appeared more abundant and predominantly cytoplasmic. Moreover the staining within the carcinomas was similar irrespective of the degree of histological differentiation, Dukes' stage or ploidy status. Also, it is worth noting that the abnormal distribution of *ras* proteins did not appear to be directly related to changes in the *ras* genes, because similar staining patterns were observed in tumours both with and without amplification or mutation of their *ras* genes.

Burmer and Loeb (1989) observed the majority of human colon carcinomas and adenomas to contain mutations of Ki-*ras* and almost exclusively in codon 12. No correlation could be made with the ploidy status of either the adenomas or carcinomas.

Thus, although there have been many reports of altered expression of p21 (Spandidos and Kerr, 1984; Thor *et al.*, 1984; Williams *et al.*, 1985; Augenlicht *et al.*, 1987; Michelassi *et al.*, 1987, 1988), until the studies of Bos *et al.* (1987) and Forrester *et al.* (1987) there was no real clue as to which member of the *ras* gene family was important. It is still not totally clear (because of the methods used) whether increased expression and mutational activation are independent events. However, if we are indeed looking at increased expression of the activated *ras* oncogene in some of these studies, variations in the level of expression do not appear to be directly related to clinically evident phenotypic differences. One thing that is abundantly clear is that *ras* gene mutations alone are not sufficient to explain the progression through the adenoma–carcinoma sequence.

As discussed in Chapter 2, another type of genetic alteration involved in colorectal carcinoma is allelic deletion of chromosome 5. The locus segregating with familial polyposis coli (FPC; or familial adenomatous polyposis, FAP) has been mapped to the long arm of chromosome 5 (Herrera *et al.*, 1986; Bodmer *et al.*, 1987; Leppert *et al.*, 1987) and approximately 20 per cent of colorectal carcinomas from patients without FPC (FAP) were reported to have allelic losses of chromosome 5 sequences (Solomon *et al.*, 1987). More recently Vogelstein *et al.* (1988) presented a highly detailed study of the genetic alterations they identified as being important in colorectal tumour development. They found *ras* gene mutations in 58 per cent of adenomas greater than 1 cm in size and in 47 per cent of carcinomas. *Ras* mutations were found in only 9 per cent of adenomas under 1 cm in size. Sequences on chromosome 5 that were linked to the gene for FPC (FAP) were not lost in adenomas from the FPC (FAP) patients, but were lost in 29 and 35 per cent of adenomas and carcinomas respectively from other patients. They also found a specific region of chromosome 18 deleted in 73 per cent of carcinomas and 47 per cent of advanced adenomas, but in only 11–13 per cent of early stage adenomas. A region of the short arm of chromosome 17 was usually lost only in carcinomas. Interestingly the *ras* gene alterations and three other alterations appeared to accumulate in a fashion that paralleled the clinical progression of the tumours (Fig. 6.2). These results were thought to be consistent with a model of colorectal tumourigenesis which involved the activation of an oncogene coupled with the loss of several genes that normally suppress malignancy.

Involvement of c-*myc* in colorectal cancer

The *myc* oncogene codes for a 62 kDa phosphoprotein localised in the nucleus which has been suggested to be involved in RNA processing (Spector *et al.*, 1987), DNA synthesis (Studzinski *et al.*, 1988) and the regulation of transcription (Kaddurah-Daouk *et al.*, 1987). In cell culture constitutively elevated expression of c-*myc* has been shown to alter both the growth factor responsiveness of the cells and their tumourigenic

Fig. 6.2. Genetic alterations during colorectal tumour progression. The percentage of tumours with the indicated genetic alteration is plotted for each type of tumour (Vogelstein *et al.*, 1988).

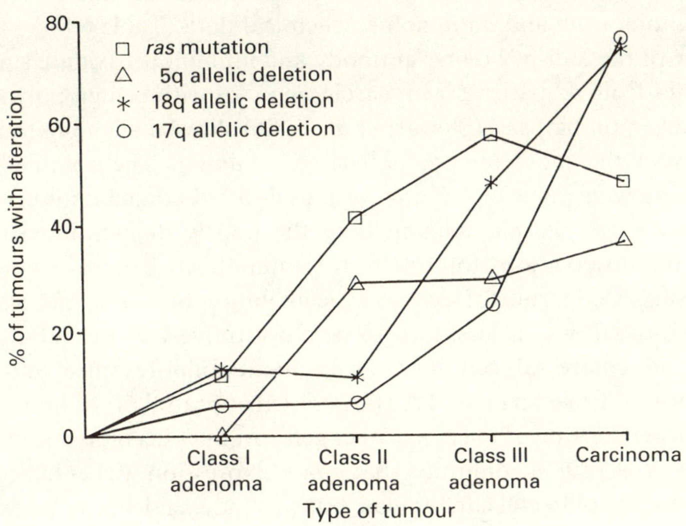

potential. However, the *myc* oncogene is probably best known for being the oncogene that cooperates with the *ras* oncogene in *in vitro* cell systems to give transformation (Land *et al.*, 1983). Elevated levels of *myc* are also known to co-exist with an activated *ras* gene in the malignant HL-60 cell line (Murray *et al.*, 1983). Erisman *et al.* (1985) showed 68 per cent of primary adenocarcinomas of the colon to exhibit elevated expression of c-*myc* which was not accompanied by amplification and rearrangement of the gene. However in a separate study (Erisman *et al.*, 1988) no correlation could be made between elevated *myc* expression, recurrence of the disease and patient survival. Calbretta *et al.* (1985), in a study of the expression of *myc* and other cell-cycle-dependent genes in colorectal carcinoma, showed the increase in expression of the c-*myc* gene to be accompanied by a parallel increase in two G_1-specific genes and an S-phase-specific gene. In a separate study of the *myb* oncogene *myc* was also shown to be increased in five out of six instances where *myb* was elevated. Elevated c-*myc* expression has also been reported in colon carcinoma cell lines in the absence of amplification (Yoshimoto *et al.*, 1986).

However, it was not until the isolation of monoclonal antibodies specific for the c-*myc* proto-oncogene product (Evan *et al.*, 1985) that the involvement of elevated *myc* in colon tumours was studied extensively. Sikora *et al.* (1987) examined c-*myc* expression in tumours and adjacent normal tissue removed during radical surgery from 15 colorectal patients using immunoblotting. Evidence for gene amplification or rearrangement was studied by DNA hybridisation and finally both normal and tumour tissue was examined immunohistochemically. Transcripts of c-*myc* mRNA were elevated in 12 out of 15 tumours and correlated well with the immunoblotting and immunohistochemical data (Table 6.8).

Use of the anti-p62 c-*myc* antibody and immunoperoxidase staining on samples from 42 patients with carcinomas, 24 with benign polyps and 15 normal colon biopsies (Stewart *et al.*, 1986) showed adenomatous polyps to reveal the most intense pattern of staining. The colonic tumours showed a wide range of staining, with well-differentiated tumours containing more cytoplasmic staining than the poorly differentiated tumours. Like the observations for *ras* from immunohistochemical studies, these data suggested a role for c-*myc* in the evolution of colonic neoplasia. The c-*myc* protein was also shown to be constitutively expressed at elevated levels in colorectal cell lines using immunofluorescence and ELISA techniques (Erisman *et al.*, 1988). A critical appraisal of the immunohistochemical detection of the c-*myc* oncogene product in colorectal carcinoma (Jones *et al.*, 1987) confirmed that c-*myc* expression was enhanced in the majority of colorectal carcinomas, but was independent of clinical behav-

Table 6.8. *c-*myc *oncogene expression in colorectal cancer (Sikhora* et al., *1987)*

Patient no.	Age	Sex	Dukes' stage	Differentiation	Immunohistology	c-*myc* mRNA	p62[c-myc]
1	65	M	B	Moderate	+ +	8	4
2	66	F	B	Poor	+	ND[a]	ND
3	83	F	B	Moderate	+ +	8	8
4	78	M	C	Moderate	+ + +	8	16
5	51	F	B	Moderate	+	2	ND
6	52	M	B	Well	+ + + +	16	32
7	59	M	B	Moderate	+ + +	8	4
8	56	F	C	Moderate	+ + +	4	ND
9	64	M	B	Well	+ + +	16	32
10	64	M	B	Well	+ + + +	8	32
11	58	M	A	Moderate	+ +	4	ND
12	70	F	C	Poor	+	2	ND
13	65	F	C	Poor	+	ND	ND
14	70	M	B	Moderate	+ + +	8	8
15	57	M	B	Poor	+ +	ND	ND

Note: [a]ND, non-detectable.

iour. Extension of these studies to non-malignant and pre-malignant gastro-intestinal disorders (Ciclitira *et al.*, 1987) showed low levels of expression of the c-*myc* oncogene product in normal colonic tissue but increased expression in inflammatory disorders including Crohn's disease and ulcerative colitis. As had previously been observed for the dysplastic areas of benign adenomas, c-*myc* expression was also increased in colonic dysplasia associated with ulcerative colitis. It seemed increasingly, therefore, that immunohistochemical quantification of c-*myc* could be used to identify the proliferative response of the colonic mucosa not only in the hyperproliferative state of neoplasia but also the proliferative response of the mucosa associated with inflammation. However, since staining is affected by fixation and processing, immunohistochemical staining on routinely processed specimens should be interpreted with caution.

It was also thought that elevated levels of c-*myc* RNA might be a marker for a distinct type of colorectal carcinoma that involves the same type of genetic events as FPC (FAP) (Rothberg, 1987), but bearing in mind all other available evidence this is likely to reflect proliferation differences. Confirmation that this might well be the case came from studies of the inhibition of cell proliferation on colon carcinoma cell lines in culture. Polyamine depletion generally results in an inhibition of cell growth and difluoromethylornithine (DFMO) depletion in colon carcinoma cells in culture resulted in a greater than 90 per cent reduction in expression of the c-*myc* proto-oncogene (Celano *et al.*, 1988). Also, transforming growth factor-β (TGF-β) is known to exhibit proliferation-inhibiting and differentiation-like effects on the colon carcinoma cell line MOSER. c-*myc* expression is repressed in response to TGF-β in the same cell line (Mulder *et al.*, 1988). Similar observations were made on colon carcinoma cell lines MOSER and HCT116 using the maturational agent *N,N*-dimethylformamide (DMF). The reduction in c-*myc* expression did not require protein synthesis and occurred only a few minutes after addition of DMF (Mulder and Brattain, 1988). More specifically proliferating, but not late log phase, MOSER cells responded to TGF-β with a repression of c-*myc* expression and inhibition of cell proliferation. Collectively these data indicate that repression of c-*myc* is associated with reduced cellular proliferation and induction of a more benign phenotype.

Over-expression of c-*myc* in colon carcinoma cell lines may drive cells to continue to proliferate despite the depletion of the serum growth factors. c-*myc* has already been shown to dictate whether a cell continues to proliferate or whether it proceeds along a given maturation pathway in an erythroleukaemic cell line (Dimitrovsky *et al.*, 1986). Thus, *myc* expression in studies involving the screening of colorectal tumours is probably a marker of the proliferation status of the cell. As *myc* is clearly regulated at the level of transcription, the significance of reports of *myc* amplification in certain cell lines is unclear (von Hoff *et al.*, 1988). Dolcetti *et al.* (1988) in a detailed study of 44 cases of colonic or rectal carcinoma showed amplification of c-*myc* in only one case and no evidence of rearrangement. This suggests that structural activation of the *myc* gene and/or amplification are unlikely to play a major role in tumour induction or tumour progression.

The role of other oncogenes

Several studies have looked at a spectrum of oncogenes at the DNA level. No rearrangement or amplification of *fos* was found (Alexander *et al.*, 1986). In another study of 45 colon carcinomas and 15 benign adenomas, amplification of c-*myc* and c-*erbB* and allelic deletion of Ha-*ras* or c-*myb* were found to be the most frequent changes (Meltzer *et al.*, 1987). Messenger RNA levels of c-*fos* were studied together with Ha-*ras*, Ki-*ras* and *myc* in 39 samples from 17 patients (Monnat *et al.*, 1987). Only 50 per cent exhibited increased levels of one or more of the four oncogenes relative to the normal mucosa. The data suggested, in fact, that the patients studied could be subdivided into two groups, one with high levels of oncogene expression and the second showing no increase in expression relative to non-involved mucosa. Follow-up of the patients showed that all deaths occurred in high expressors, suggesting a correlation between high expression and aggressiveness of the disease. The tyrosine-specific protein kinase activity of pp60src is also known to be elevated in colon tumour cell lines compared with normal mucosa cells (Bolen *et al.*, 1987). The *trk* transforming gene has also been identified in colon carcinoma (Mitra *et al.*, 1987). The c-*erbB* oncogene has been shown to be amplified in a colon adenocarcinoma (Yokota *et al.*, 1986). High levels of c-*myb* proto-oncogene expression have been reported in six out of ten subjects affected by colon carcinoma when compared with normal mucosa (Torelli *et al.*, 1987) and in five out of six of these cases the mRNA levels of c-*myc*, histone h3 and ODC mRNAs were also increased, suggesting that there is a relationship between the high expression of c-*myb* and the fraction of cycling cells. The transforming gene *hst* was identified in the NIH3T3 cell system as being responsible for the transforming activity in one colon carcinoma cell line. An amplified *myb* oncogene has also been reported in a colon carcinoma cell line (Winquist *et al.*, 1985).

Multiple genetic steps involved in the development of the disease

From the studies cited above it can be concluded that mutated *ras* genes are important in the early stages of tumour development. Approximately 50 per cent of carcinomas (Bos *et al.*, 1987; Forrester *et al.*, 1987) and 50 per cent of adenomas of greater than 1 cm in size (Vogelstein *et al.*, 1988; Boughdady, Schofield and Kinsella, unpublished observations) contain *ras* gene mutations. *Ras* gene mutations may therefore be the initiating event in a subset of colorectal tumours. Also, adenomas with *ras* gene mutations may be more likely to progress to carcinomas than those without (Fearon and Vogelstein, 1990). The role for the *myc* oncogene is less clear and its increased expression is probably quite simply a consequence of increased cell turnover.

As mentioned in Chapter 5 and earlier in this chapter, the loss of specific chromosomal regions is a common occurrence in colorectal neoplasia. Such allelic losses in other tumours have been interpreted as evidence that the specific regions involved contain tumour suppressor genes which regulate cell growth and differentiation and suppress tumour formation (Cavenee *et al.*, 1983; Knudson, 1985; Seizinger *et al.*, 1987). Cytogenetic and linkage studies have mapped the locus for FPC (FAP), which confers an inherited predisposition to colorectal carcinoma on the individuals affected, to chromosome 5q (Bodmer *et al.*, 1987; Leppert *et al.*, 1987). In patients without FPC (FAP), allelic losses of chromosome 5q have been observed in 20–50 per cent of colorectal carcinomas and 30 per cent of adenomas (Vogelstein *et al.*, 1988; Sasaki *et al.*, 1989). However, in adenomas from patients with FPC (FAP), allelic losses of chromosome 5q are rare, suggesting a mutation at this locus in these patients (Solomon *et al.*, 1987; Vogelstein *et al.*, 1988; Sasaki *et al.*, 1989). Interestingly, a candidate tumour suppressor gene which mapped to chromosome region 5q21 and was mutated in three sporadic colorectal tumours was proposed as a candidate gene for the inherited defect FPC (FAP) (Kinzler *et al.*, 1991*a*). However this gene, *MCC* (mutated in colorectal cancer), was later found not to be mutated in FPC (FAP) patients (Nishisho *et al.*, 1991). The latest colorectal tumour suppressor gene to be identified also maps to chromosome region 5q21 and is believed to be the gene for FPC (FAP) (Kinzler *et al.*, 1991*b*; Nishisho *et al.*, 1991; Groden *et al.*, 1991; Joslyn *et al.*, 1991). Mutations in this gene, designated *APC* (adenomatous polyposis coli) or *FAP*, have been shown to occur in FPC (FAP) patients and in sporadic colorectal tumours.

The loss of chromosome 17p has been observed in 75 per cent of colorectal tumours examined (Vogelstein *et al.*, 1988; Delattre *et al.*, 1989), but is relatively rare in adenomas at any stage (Figs. 5.1 and 6.2; Vogelstein *et al.*, 1988; Fearon and Vogelstein, 1990). The specific region of chromosome loss on chromosome 17p is also common to other tumours and has been found to contain the p53 gene, which is now known to be a tumour suppressor gene and not an oncogene as previously supposed (Baker *et al.*, 1989). Mutations in the remaining p53 genes have been observed in several colorectal tumours that have a concomitant loss of their other p53 allele (Baker *et al.*, 1989; Nigro *et al.*, 1989). Thus, in colorectal tumours a mutation in one allele is commonly associated with the loss of the remaining wild-type allele. This is consistent with the thesis that the wild-type p53 gene acts to inhibit tumour formation.

The loss of a portion of chromosome 18q is seen in approximately 70 per cent of colorectal tumours and in almost 50 per cent of late adenomas (Fig. 6.2; Vogelstein *et al.*, 1988). This region of chromosome 18 contains a candidate tumour suppressor gene *DCC* (deleted in colorectal carcinoma), the gene product of which is related to a family of cell adhesion molecules and the expression of which is reduced or absent in colorectal tumours (Fearon *et al.*, 1990; Fearon and Vogelstein, 1990). Thus, any reduction in expression might lead to a diminution of the growth-restraining signals associated with such adhesion.

As a consequence of these molecular observations, Vogelstein and coworkers have proposed a model (Fig. 6.3) for the development of colorectal carcinoma that involves at least four distinct classes of genetic event: (1) the mutation or deletion of a gene on chromosome 5q, (2) a *ras* gene mutation, (3) a deletion or mutation of the *DCC* gene on chromosome 18q, and (4) a deletion and mutation of the p53 gene on chromosome 17p. However, as a subset of the allelic losses is likely to demonstrate a mutation in the retained allele, it seems likely that some of the molecular events described above will actually be shown to involve two independent genetic events. Thus, a model involving only four or five clear genetic stages is probably extremely conservative. Other allelic losses have been observed in colorectal tumours (Fig. 5.2) and most colorectal carcinomas have at least one other allelic loss in addition to those on 5q, 17p and 18q. It has been suggested that an epigenetic event such as hypomethylation might contribute to genomic instability and influence the rate of allelic loss.

What is certain, however, is that the genetic alterations underlying colorectal tumourigenesis involve the action of at least one activated, dominantly acting oncogene coupled to the loss or mutation of several growth-regulating or tumour suppressor genes. Certainly the introduction of normal chromosome 5 or 18 has been shown to suppress the tumourigenicity of a human carcinoma cell line *in vitro* (Tanaka *et al.*, 1991). Also, although the usual order of events is that seen in Fig. 6.3 it is the accumulation rather than the precise order of events that is important

Fig. 6.3. A genetic model for colorectal tumourigenesis (Fearon and Vogelstein, 1990).

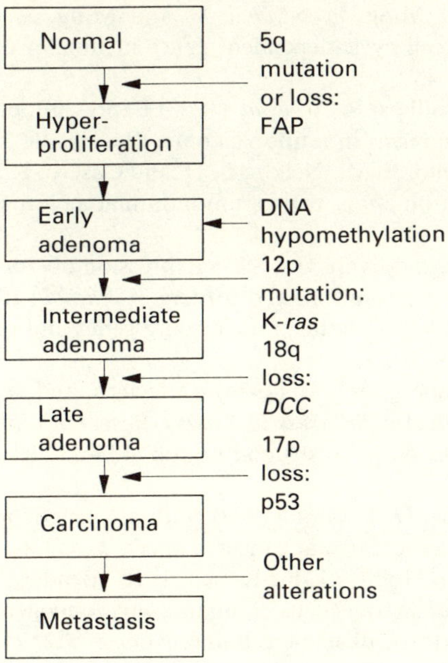

(Fearon and Vogelstein, 1990). The application of this molecular knowledge to diagnosis and screening for the disease will be addressed in Chapter 8. After all, the disease is totally preventable if detected before the carcinoma stage.

References

Alexander, R. J., Buxbaum, J. N. and Raicht, R. F. (1986) Oncogene alterations in primary human colon tumours. *Gastroenterology*, **91**, 1503–10.

Augenlicht, L. H., Augeron, C., Yander, G. and Laboisse, C. (1987) Overexpression of *ras* in mucus-secreting human colon carcinoma cells of low tumourigenicity. *Cancer Res.*, **47**, 3763–5.

Baker, S. J., Fearon, E. R., Nigro, J. M., *et al.* (1989) Chromosome 17 deletions and p53 gene mutations in colorectal carcinomas. *Science*, **244**, 217–21.

Bishop, J. M. (1983) Cellular oncogenes and retroviruses. *Annu. Rev. Biochem.*, **52**, 301–54.

Bodmer, W. F., Bailey, C. J., Bodmer, J., *et al.* (1987) Localization of the gene for familial adenomatous polyposis on chromsome 5. *Nature*, **328**, 614–16.

Bolen, J. B., Veilette, A., Schwartz, A. M., Deseau, V. and Rosen, N. (1987) Analysis of pp60src in human colon carcinoma and normal human colon mucosal cells. *Oncogene Res.*, **1**, 149–68.

Bos, J., Fearon, E. R., Hamilton, S. R., Verlaan-de-Vries, M., van Boom, J. H., van der Eb, A. J. and Vogelstein, B. (1987) Prevalence of *ras* gene mutations in human colorectal cancers. *Nature*, **327**, 293.

Burmer, G. C. and Loeb, L. A. (1989) Mutations in the K-*ras* 2 oncogene during progressive stages of human colon carcinoma. *Proc. Natl. Acad. Sci. USA*, **85**, 2403–7.

Calabretta, B., Kaczmarek, L., Ming, P. N., Au, F. and Ming, S. C. (1985) Expressing c-*myc* and other cell cycle-dependent genes in human colon neoplasia. *Cancer Res.*, **45**, 6000–4.

Cavenee, W. K., Dryja, T. P., Phillips, R. A., *et al.* (1983) Expression of recessive alleles by chromosomal mechanisms in retinoblastoma. *Nature*, **305**, 779–84.

Celano, P., Baylin, S. B., Giardello, F. M., Nelkin, B. D. and Casero, R. A. (1988) Effect of polyamine depletion on c-*myc* expression in human colon carcinoma cells. *J. Biol. Chem.*, **263**, 5491–4.

Ciclitira, P. J., MaCartney, J. C. and Evan, G. (1987) Expression of c-*myc* in non-malignant and pre-malignant gastrointestinal disorders. *J. Pathol.*, **151**, 293–6.

Cooper, G. M. and Lane, M. (1984) Cellular transforming genes and oncogenes. *Biochim. Biophys. Acta*, **738**, 9–20.

Cunningham, J. M. and Weinberg, R. A. (1984) Detection and analysis of oncogenes in colon carcinoma. In: *Progress in Cancer Research and Therapy*, vol. 29, ed. S. R. Wolman and A. J. Mastromarino, pp. 403–11. Raven Press, New York.

Delattre, P., Olschwang, S., Law, D. J., *et al.* (1989) Multiple genetic alterations distinguish distal from proximal colorectal cancer. *Lancet*, **2**, 353–6.

Dimitrovsky, E., Kuehl, W. M., Hollis, G. F., Kirsch, I. R., Bender, T. P. and Segal, S. (1986) Expression of a transfected human c-*myc* oncogene inhibits differentiation of a mouse erythroleukaemic cell line. *Nature*, **322**, 748–50.

Dolcetti, R., De Re, V., Viel, A., Pistello, M., Tavian, M. and Boiocchi, M. (1988) Nuclear oncogene amplification or rearrangement is not involved in human colorectal malignancies. *Eur. J. Cancer Clin. Oncol.*, **24**, 1321–8.

Erisman, M. D., Litwin, S., Keidan, R. D., Comis, R. L. and Astrin, S. M. (1985) Non-correlation of the expression of the c-*myc* oncogene in colorectal carcinoma with recurrence of disease or patient survival. *Cancer Res.*, **48**, 1350–5.

Erisman, M. D., Rothberg, P. G., Diehl, R. E., Morse, C. C., Spandorfer, J. M. and Astrin, S. M. (1988) Deregulation of c-*myc* gene expression in human colon carcinoma is not accompanied by amplification or rearrangement of the gene. *Mol. Cell Biol.*, **5**, 1969–76.

Evan, G., Lewis, C. K., Ramsey, G. and Bishop, J. M. (1985) Isolation of monoclonal antibodies specific for the human c-*myc* proto-oncogene product. *Mol. Cell Biol.*, **5**, 3610–16.

Fearon, E. R. and Vogelstein, B. (1990) A genetic model for colorectal tumourigenesis. *Cell*, **61**, 759–67.

Fearon, E. R., Cho, K. R., Nigro, J. M., *et al.* (1990) Identification of a chromosome 18q gene that is altered in colorectal cancers. *Science*, **247**, 49–56.

Feinberg, A. P., Vogelstein, B., Droller, M. J., Banghin, S. B. and Nelkin, B. D. (1983) Mutation affecting the 12th amino acid of the c-Ha-*ras* oncogene product occurs infrequently in human cancer. *Science*, **220**, 1175–7.

Forrester, K., Almoguera, C., Han, K., Grizzle, W. E. and Perucho, M. (1987) Detection of high incidence of K-*ras* oncogenes during human colon tumourigenesis. *Nature*, **327**, 298–303.

Furth, M. E., Davis, L. J., Fleurdelys, B. and Scolnick, E. M. (1982) Monoclonal antibodies to the p21 products of the transforming gene of Ha-MuSV and of the cellular *ras* gene family. *J. Virol.*, **43**, 294–304.

Gallick, G. E., Kurzrock, R., Kloetzer, W. S., Arlinghaus, R. B. and Gutterman, J. U. (1985) Expression of p21 *ras* in fresh primary and metastatic human colorectal tumours. *Proc. Natl. Acad. Sci. USA*, **82**, 1795–9.

Gibbs, J. B., Sigal, I. S., Poe, M. and Scolnick, E. M. (1984) Intrinsic GTPase activity distinguishes normal and oncogenic *ras* p21 molecules. *Proc. Natl. Acad. Sci. USA*, **81**, 5704–8.

Greenhalgh, D. A. and Kinsella, A. R. (1985) c-Ha-*ras* not c-Ki-*ras* involvement in colorectal carcinoma. *Carcinogenesis*, **6**, 1533–5.

Groden, J., Thilveris, A., Samowitz, W., *et al.* (1991) Identification and characterisation of familial adenomatous polyposis gene. *Cell*, **66**, 589–600.

Herrera, L., Kakati, S., Gibas, L., Pietrzak, E. and Sandberg, A. A. (1986) Brief clinical report: Gardner syndrome in a man with an interstitial deletion of 5p. *Am. J. Med. Genet.*, **25**, 473–6.

Horan Hand, P., Thor, A., Wunderlich, D., Muraro, R., Caruso, A. and Schlom, J. (1984) Monoclonal antibodies of pre-defined specificity detect activated *ras* gene expression in human mammary and colon carcinomas. *Proc. Natl. Acad. Sci. USA*, **81**, 5227–31.

Jones, D. J., Ghosh, A. K., Moore, M. and Schofield, P. F. (1987) A critical appraisal of the immuno-histochemical detection of the c-*myc* oncogene product in colorectal cancer. *Br. J. Cancer*, **56**, 779–83.

Joslyn, G., Carlson, M., Thilveris, A., *et al.* (1991) Identification of deletion mutations and three new genes at the familial polyposis locus. *Cell*, **66**, 601–13.

Kaddurah-Daouk, R., Greene, J. M., Baldwin, A. S. and Kingston, R. E. (1987) Activation and repression of mammalian gene expression by the c-*myc* protein. *Genes Dev.*, **1**, 347–57.

Kamata, T. and Feramisco, J. R. (1984) Epidermal growth factor stimulates guanine nucleotide binding activity and phosphorylation of *ras* oncogene proteins. *Nature*, **310**, 147–50.

Kerr, I. B., Lee, F. D., Quintanilla, M. and Balmain, A. (1985) Immunocytochemical demonstration of p21 *ras* family oncogene product in normal mucosa and in malignant and pre-malignant tumours of the colorectum. *Br. J. Cancer*, **52**, 695–700.

Kinzler, K. W., Nilbert, M. C., Vogelstein, B., *et al.* (1991*a*) Identification of a gene located at chromosome 5q21 that is mutated in colorectal cancers. *Science*, **251**, 1366–70.

Kinzler, K. W., Nilbert, M. C., Su, L. K., *et al.* (1991*b*) Identification of FAP locus genes from chromosome 5q21. *Science*, **253**, 661–5.

Knudson, A. G. (1985) Hereditary cancer, oncogenes and anti-oncogenes. *Cancer Res.*, **45**, 1437–43.

Koda, T., Sasaki, A., Matsushima, S. and Kakinuma, M. (1987) A transforming gene *hst* found in NIH3T3 cells transformed with DNA from three stomach cancers and a colon cancer. *Jpn. J. Cancer Res.*, **78**, 325–8.

Land, H., Parada, L. F. and Weinberg, R. A. (1983) Tumourigenic conversion of primary embryo fibroblasts requires at least two co-operating oncogenes. *Nature*, **304**, 596–602.

Leppert, M., Dobbs, M., Scrambler, P., *et al.* (1987) The gene for familial polyposis coli maps to the long arm of chromosome 5. *Science*, **238**, 1411–13.

McCoy, M. S., Toole, J., Cunningham, J. M., Chang, E. H., Lowy, D. R. and Weinberg, R. A. (1983) Characterisation of a human colon/lung carcinoma oncogene. *Nature*, **302**, 79–81.

McGrath, J. P., Capon, D. J., Goeddel, D. V. and Levinson, A. D. (1984) Comparative biochemical properties of normal and activated human *ras* p21 protein. *Nature*, **310**, 644.

Meltzer, S. J., Ahnen, D. J., Battifora, H., *et al.* (1987) Proto-oncogene abnormalities in colon cancers and adenomatous polyps. *Gastroenterology*, **92**, 1174–80.

Michelassi, F., Leuthner, S., Lubienski, M., Bostwick, D., Rodgers, J., Handcock, M. and Block, G. E. (1987) *Ras* oncogene p21 levels parallel malignant potential of different human colonic benign conditions. *Arch. Surg.*, **122**, 141–6.

Michelassi, F., Vannucci, L., Montag, A., Chappele, R., Rodgers, J. and Block, G. E. (1988) *Ras* oncogene expression as a prognostic indicator of rectal adenocarcinoma. *J. Surg. Res.*, **45**, 15–20.

Mitra, G., Martin-Zanca, D. and Barbacid, M. (1987) Identification of p70trk product of the human *trk* oncogene. *Proc. Natl. Acad. Sci. USA*, **84**, 6707–11.

Monnat, M., Tardy, S., Saraga, P., Diggelman, H. and Costa, J. (1987) Prognostic implications of expression of the cellular genes *myc*, *fos*, Ha-*ras* and Ki-*ras* in colon carcinoma. *Int. J. Cancer*, **40**, 293–9.

Mulder, K. M. and Brattain, M. G. (1988) Alterations in c-*myc* expression in relation to maturational status of human colon carcinoma cells. *Int. J. Cancer*, **42**, 64–70.

Mulder, K. M., Levine, A. E., Hernandez, X., McKnight, M. K., Brattain, D. E.

and Brattain, M. G. (1988) Modulation of c-*myc* by transforming growth factor-β in human colon carcinoma cells. *Biochem. Biophys. Res. Commun.*, **150**, 711–16.

Murray, M. S., Cunningham, J. M., Parada, L. F., *et al.* (1983) The HL-60 transforming sequence: a *ras* oncogene co-existing with altered *myc* genes in haemopoietic tumours. *Cell*, **33**, 744–57.

Nigro, J. M., Baker, S. J., Preisinger, A. C., *et al.* (1989) Mutations in the p53 gene occur in diverse tumour types. *Nature*, **342**, 705–7.

Nishisho, I., Nakamura, Y., Miyoshi, Y., *et al.* (1991) Mutations of chromosome 5q21 genes in FAP and colorectal cancer patients. *Science*, **253**, 665–9.

Nitta, N., Ochiai, M., Nagao, M. and Sugimura, T. (1987) Amino acid substitution at codon 13 of the N-*ras* oncogene in rectal cancer in a Japanese patient. *Jpn. J. Cancer Res.*, **78**, 21–6.

Perucho, M., Goldfarb, M., Shimizu, K., *et al.* (1981) Human tumour-derived cell lines contain common and different transforming genes. *Cell*, **27**, 467–76.

Pulciani, S., Santos, E., Lauver, A. V., *et al.* (1982) Oncogenes in human tumour cell lines: molecular cloning of a transforming gene from human bladder carcinoma cells. *Proc. Natl. Acad. Sci. USA*, **79**, 2845–9.

Robinson, A., Williams, A. R. W., Piris, J., *et al.* (1986) Evaluation of monoclonal antibody to *ras* peptide, RAP-5, claimed to bind preferentially to cells of infiltrating carcinomas. *Br. J. Cancer*, **54**, 877–83.

Rothberg, P. G. (1987) The role of the oncogene c-*myc* in sporadic large bowel cancer and familial polyposis coli. *Semin. Surg. Oncol.*, **3**, 152–8.

Salhab, N., Jones, D. J., Bos, J. L., Kinsella, A. and Schofield, P. F. (1989) The detection of *ras* gene alterations and *ras* proteins in colorectal cancer. *Dis. Colon Rectum*, **32**, 659–64.

Sasaki, M., Okamoto, M., Sato, C., *et al.* (1989) Loss of constitutional heterozygosity in colorectal tumours from patients with familial polyposis coli and those with non-polyposis colorectal carcinoma. *Cancer Res.*, **49**, 4402–6.

Seizinger, B. R., Rouleau, G., Ozelius, L. J., *et al.* (1987) Common pathogenic mechanism for three tumour types in bilateral acoustic neurofibromatosis. *Science*, **236**, 317–19.

Shih, T. Y. (1984) Oncogenes and cancer: the p21 *ras* genes. *Cancer Invest.*, **2**, 109–23.

Sikora, K., Chan, S., Evans, G., *et al.* (1987) c-*myc* oncogene expression in colorectal cancer. *Cancer Res.*, **59**, 1289–95.

Slattery, M. L., Sorenson, A. W., Mahoney, A. W., French, T. K., Kritchevsky, D. and Street, J. C. (1988) Diet and colon cancer: assessment of risk by fiber type and food source. *J. Natl. Cancer Inst.*, **80**, 1474–80.

Solomon, E., Voss, R., Hall, V., *et al.* (1987) Chromosome 5 allele loss in human colorectal carcinomas. *Nature*, **328**, 616–19.

Spandidos, D. A. and Kerr, I. B. (1984) Elevated expression of the human *ras* oncogene family in premalignant and malignant tumours of the colorectum. *Br. J. Cancer*, **49**, 681–8.

Spandidos, D. A., Harrison, P. R. and Paul, J. (1981) Transfer and expression of herpes simplex virus thymidine kinase and human globin genes in mammalian cells studied by spot hybridisation assays. *Biosci. Rep.*, **1**, 911–20.

Spector, D. L., Watt, R. A. and Sullivan, N. F. (1987) The v-*myc* and c-*myc* oncogene proteins co-localise *in situ* with small nuclear ribonucleoprotein particles. *Oncogene*, **1**, 5–12.

Stewart, J., Evan, G., Watson, J. and Sikora, K. (1986) Detection of the c-*myc* oncogene product in colonic polyps and carcinomas. *Br. J. Cancer*, **53**, 1–6.

Studzinski, G. P., Brelvi, Z. S., Feldman, S. C. and Watt, R. A. (1986) Participation of c-*myc* protein in DNA synthesis of human cells. *Science*, **234**, 467–70.

Sweet, R. W., Yokoyama, S., Kamata, T., Feramisco, J. R., Rosenberg, M. and Gross, M. (1984) The product of *ras* is a GTPase and the T24 oncogene mutant is deficient in this activity. *Nature*, **311**, 273–5.

Tanaka, K., Oshimura, M., Kikuchi, R., *et al.* (1991) Suppression of tumourigenicity in human colon carcinoma cells by introduction of normal chromosome 5 or 18. *Nature*, **349**, 340–2.

Thor, A., Horan Hand, P., Wunderlich, D., Caruso, A., Muraro, R. and Schlom, J. (1984) Monoclonal antibodies define differential *ras* gene expression in differential and benign colonic diseases. *Nature*, **311**, 562–5.

Torelli, G., Venturelli, D., Colo, A., *et al.* (1987) Expression of the c-*myc* proto-oncogene and other cell cycle-related genes in normal and neoplastic colonic mucosa. *Cancer Res.*, **47**, 5266–9.

Vogelstein, B., Fearon, E. R., Hamilton, S. R., *et al.* (1988) Genetic alterations during colorectal tumour development. *New Engl. J. Med.*, **319**, 525–32.

Von Hoff, D. D., Needham-van Devanter, D. R., Yucel, J., Windle, B. E. and Wahl, G. M. (1988) Amplified human *myc* genes localised to submicroscopic circular DNA molecules. *Proc. Natl. Acad. Sci. USA*, **85**, 4804–8.

Williams, A. R. W., Piris, J., Spandidos, D. A. and Wyllie, A. H. (1985) Immunohistochemical detection of the *ras* oncogene p21 product in an experimental tumour and in human colorectal neoplasms. *Br. J. Cancer*, **52**, 687–93.

Winquist, R., Knuutila, S., Leprince, D., Stehlin, D. and Alitalo, K. (1985) Mapping of amplified c-*myc* oncogene, sister chromatid exchanges and karyotypic analysis of the colo 205 colon carcinoma cell line. *Cancer Genet. Cytogenet.*, **18**, 251–64.

Yokota, J., Tsunetsugu-Yokota, Y., Battifora, H., Lefevre, C. and Cline, M. J. (1980) Alterations in *myc*, *myb* and *ras*-Ha proto-oncogenes in cancers are frequent and show clinical correlation. *Science*, **231**, 261–5.

Yoshimoto, K., Hirohashi, S. and Sekiya, T. (1986) Increased expression of c-*myc* gene without gene amplification in human lung cancer and colon cell lines. *Jpn. J. Cancer Res.*, **77**, 540–5.

7

Principles of prevention and treatment
by P. F. Schofield

Clinicians share the curiosity of scientists about the causation of colorectal cancer but their overriding interest leans towards prevention and treatment of these diseases. Prevention is by the identification of those large bowel diseases which predispose to malignancy. Treatment relies for its best results on being undertaken when the malignant process is still localised. It is widely believed that this may be achieved by 'early' diagnosis but, as yet, there is little or no proof that early diagnosis does modify survival.

Early diagnosis is a clinical concept to describe a small, clinically detectable lesion, yet the tumour will have been present at the cellular level for months or years. It has been estimated that about 36 doublings are required before a neoplasm can be diagnosed by any investigatory method (Hunter, 1989). Some tumours have biological characteristics which predispose to very early dissemination whereas others do not. The first group will not be controlled after 'early' diagnosis because treatment will be too late. The second group will be controlled whether treated early or late, except for the few tumours that become aggressive immediately before clinical presentation. Most colorectal carcinomas belong to the second group because they develop from a benign tumour and are susceptible to diagnosis by colonoscopy. How much difference in survival could be achieved by diagnosis at the asymptomatic stage is unknown and will be discussed later.

Clinico-pathological factors

Chapters 1 and 2 have dealt with the current perceptions of the genesis of colorectal disease and its spread in humans. Nevertheless, before

Table 7.1. *Risk factors for colorectal carcinoma (CRC)*

	Approximate % of CRC patients
Previous colorectal tumour	4–5
First degree relatives with CRC	15–20
Cancer family syndrome	4–5
Familial adenomatous polyposis (FAP)	0.2
Long-standing ulcerative colitis	0.6
Increasing age only	75–80

considering screening to diagnose adenomas or carcinomas it is important to establish the natural history. The usual method of development of large bowel cancer is by malignant change in an adenoma even though the vast majority of adenomas remain benign. Malignancy is rare in small tubular adenomas but becomes progressively commoner with increasing size or in villous adenomas (Morson, 1974). There is certainly evidence that some colorectal carcinomas develop from flat lesions without a preceding raised adenoma; the frequency of this type of development is unknown, though it is believed to be relatively uncommon (Jass, 1989).

Adenomas may be symptomatic, and in particular they may produce bleeding. Under these circumstances investigation by colonoscopy should be undertaken, when it is usual to be able to remove the symptomatic adenoma or adenomas endoscopically and thus prevent malignant transformation. From the clinician's point of view it is important to recognise that colonic bleeding is an indication for colonoscopy rather than barium enema (Thoeni and Menuck, 1977). Radio-opaque contrast studies are less good methods for displaying adenomatous polyps and may show coincident unrelated disease, in particular diverticular disease. It should be noted that diverticular disease is not a cause of minor colorectal bleeding but the presence of diverticula make the interpretation of a barium enema more complicated. Our experience agrees with that of others that colonoscopy in patients with diverticular disease and bleeding always reveals a cause other than the diverticular disease, usually an adenoma (Knoepp and McCulloch, 1978).

Population surveillance

High-risk groups (Table 7.1)

The majority of patients with adenomas do not present with clinical symptoms, so we are left with the question as to how patients should be selected for assessment by colonoscopy. Family history gives us a good key to the assessment of individual risk. An interesting study showed that if only one first degree relative (parent, sibling or child) had colorectal cancer then there was no increased risk, but if there were two first degree relatives affected then there was increased risk (Grossman and Milos, 1988). This allows the recognition of a high-risk group in which regular colonoscopic survey can be advised. It is desirable to carry out a family investigation based on all patients presenting with colorectal carcinoma. There are some very obvious cancer families (see Chapter 2) and the healthy members of such families should be offered regular colonoscopy. When the association is less clear, it is less certain how justified a colonoscopic screening programme would be.

Diseases that produce increased risk of malignancy – familial polyposis coli (FPC, or familial adenomatous polyposis (FAP)), ulcerative colitis and Crohn's disease – are numerically a very minor part of the problem of prevention, but clear strategies are agreed. Patients with a family history of FPC (FAP) need to be regularly screened by colonoscopy and screening is assisted by fundoscopy to observe the congenital hypertrophy of the retinal pigmented epithelium (CHIRPE) (Blair and Trempe, 1980). Although the characteristic 5q gene deletion may come to play a part in screening, it is necessary to wait for the development of the adenomatous polyps before advising surgery. If the disease develops, there is no doubt that malignancy will occur within a decade if surgery is withheld. Historically, the operations have either been protocolectomy with ileostomy or total colectomy with ileorectal anastomosis and regular rectal surveillance (Fig. 7.1a and b). In recent years the preferred option has been total colectomy with ileal reservoir and ileo-anal anastomosis (Fig. 7.1c). Inflammatory bowel disease carries an increased risk when there is total large bowel involvement which has been present for at least 10 years. The risk is relatively greater in ulcerative colitis than in Crohn's disease. If these patients are satisfactorily managed medically then after 10 years of disease they should be placed on a surveillance programme in which colonoscopy is carried out at regular intervals with multiple biopsies. If a biopsy shows severe dysplasia or actual tumour formation there is an indication for surgery. The operative procedures in ulcerative colitis are similar to those for FPC (FAP).

Other high-risk groups include patients with bilharzial colonic polyps and uretero-colonic anastomosis, but both of these conditions are extremely rare in the UK.

Fig. 7.1. Operations for FPC (FAP) or ulcerative colitis. The broken outline indicates the area removed. (*a*) Total colectomy with ileo-rectal anastomosis. The whole of the large bowel down to but not including the rectum is removed and the small bowel at A is joined to the rectum at B. (*b*) Proctocolectomy with ileostomy. The whole of the large bowel including the anorectum is removed and the cut end of the small bowel at A is brought through the abdominal wall as an ileostomy. (*c*) Proctocolectomy, ileal reservoir plus ileo-anal anastomosis. The whole of the large bowel, including the rectum, is removed; a container for faeces (an ileal reservoir) is made out of small bowel. The segment of small bowel (A*) is sewn to make the reservoir, which is then sewn to the anus.

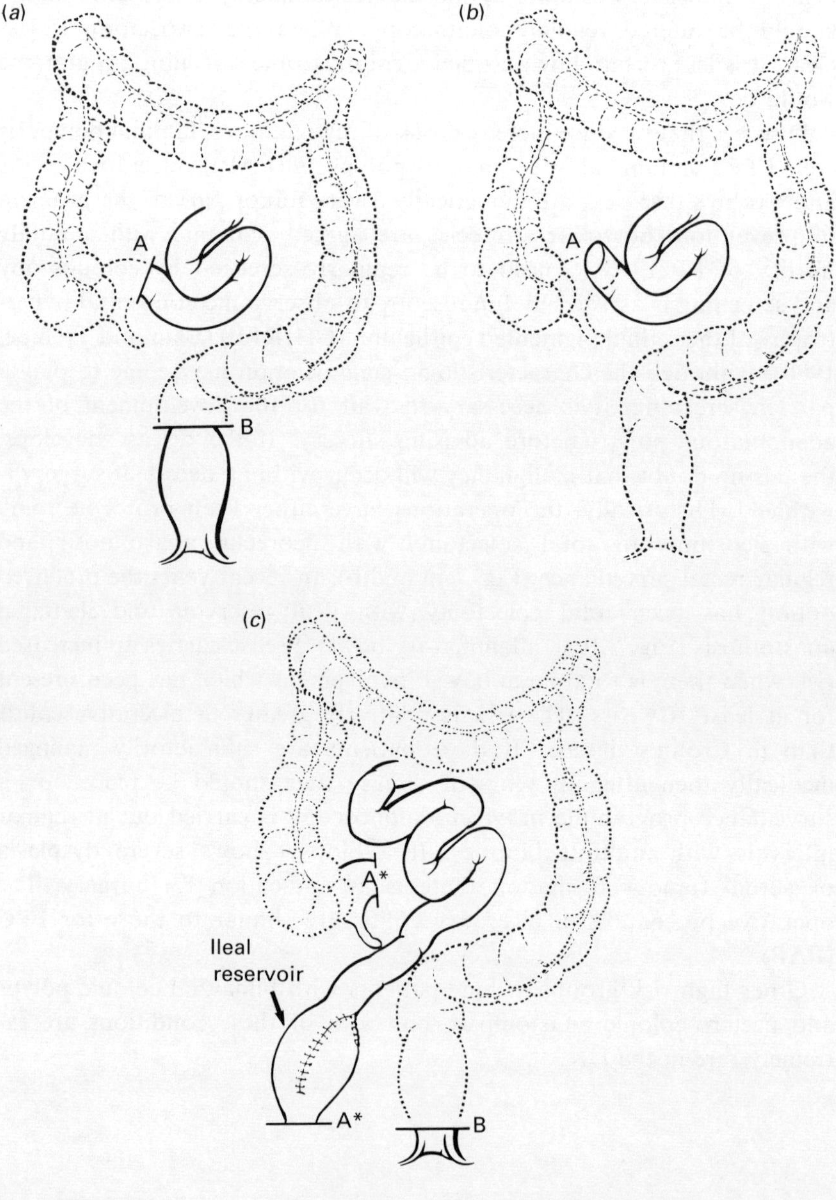

Low-risk groups

The concept of the high-risk group based on family history has already been discussed. These patients tend to be younger and form a group which requires regular colonoscopy from about the age of 40 (Itoh *et al.*, 1990). The majority of patients who develop colorectal carcinoma have no discernible risk factors; we therefore have to address the question of whether population screening is feasible and allows for earlier diagnosis.

Feasibility of screening

The incidence of colorectal carcinoma increases with age up to the seventh or eighth decade but has a relatively low prevalence below the age of 50 years (Schofield, 1990). It would seem that it is not essential to screen people below that age and certainly screening below that age would be very cost-ineffective in the absence of a strong family history. The crucial test is colonoscopy, annually if polyps are present and removed but less frequently if the colon is clear. Some individuals specifically request a regular health check programme and, in my view, colonoscopy should be introduced to such programmes starting at the age of 50–55. It has to be remembered that the procedure does carry slight hazard (a significant complication rate of about 0.1 per cent) and this has to be balanced against the possible advantage (cancer detection rate of about 0.1 per cent). Whilst in the UK, where at present health check programmes cover relatively small numbers, the incorporation of colonoscopy would be practicable, if the number of patients for health check programmes became very large then regular colonoscopy would not be feasible.

This brings us to the difficult problem of population screening. Total colonoscopy involves prior bowel preparation and in expert hands the examination takes about 30 minutes. It is obviously impracticable to carry out colonoscopy on every patient above the age of 50 – approximately 15 million in Great Britain. There has to be some simple preliminary test to select patients for colonoscopy, such as an assessment of some abnormal substance in the blood or faeces. Some years ago a reawakened fetal antigen, carcinoembryonic antigen (CEA), was found to be elevated in the serum of patients with colorectal carcinoma (Gold and Freedman, 1965). The early hopes of CEA as a reliable marker were not fulfilled because it is elevated in many other conditions and not always elevated in colorectal carcinoma. CEA has found a place in post-operative surveillance because elevation of serum levels may precede and predict clinical recurrence. Other serum markers have been found but none is sufficiently specific (Moore *et al.*, 1989).

Currently, the usual screening tests depend upon the assessment of occult blood in the faeces. This type of test is easy to perform but it is far from perfect because of varying sensitivity and specificity between the available tests. If the test is very sensitive, it identifies many people without disease and causes an unacceptably high colonoscopy load. Some tests are so sensitive that they will pick up blood derived from brushing the teeth. If the test is less sensitive it tends to miss carcinomas. It should be remembered that adenomas often do not bleed and it is particularly desirable to pick up large adenomas. In studies of asymptomatic subjects there are more adenomas and carcinomas found in patients who have positive occult blood tests but adenomas and carcinomas are also found in patients in whom the occult blood test is negative (Bertario *et al.*, 1988). Nevertheless, faecal occult bleeding does define a higher risk group and the ease of the test makes it a useful screening tool in large studies.

Although there are many tests available, the most popular compromise has been to use the Hemoccult test. The test is carried out on three or six successive days and colonoscopy is performed if any of these tests for blood is positive. The tests are more specific if the patient is on a meat-free diet and this adds to the difficulty with patient compliance in a large screening programme. In the UK it has been shown that the best way to get patient compliance is to issue invitations through General Practitioners, but even with this method it is difficult to get compliance greater than 70 per cent (Pye *et al.*, 1988). In general, compliance is approximately 50 per cent, test positivity 3 per cent and the yield about one cancer per 1000 persons screened (Ahlquist, 1990).

Efficacy of screening

Population screening based on occult-blood-directed colonoscopy has been carried out for some years, and reports from the USA (Mandel *et al.*, 1989), Denmark (Kronberg *et al.*, 1987) and the UK (Hardcastle and Pye, 1989) suggest that carcinomas are found at an earlier Dukes' stage. The most comprehensive study comes from Nottingham, England (Hardcastle *et al.*, 1989). This study includes over 100 000 subjects and compares a screened group with a non-screened group. There is no doubt that the screened patients have a higher incidence of Dukes' A carcinoma than those diagnosed in the non-screened group. However there is no evidence as yet of improved survival in the screened patients. Herein lies the problem. Does a screen-detected Dukes' A carcinoma have the same biological behaviour as a symptomatic Dukes' A carcinoma? The only study suggesting a survival advantage for screening is a small non-randomised study from Japan (Fujita *et al.*, 1990). It is only by long-term randomised studies of the Nottingham type that the question of benefit can be properly resolved.

Early clinical diagnosis

It is important that the public should be aware of the symptoms of large bowel cancer and not ignore symptoms, in particular bleeding, changing bowel habit, weight loss and anaemia. It is equally important that the physicians in primary care and in hospital practice should take these symptoms seriously. Rectal cancer usually presents with rectal bleeding and the tumour can often be felt by digital examination of the rectum, but this examination may be omitted because it is embarrassing to the patient and sometimes to the doctor. A majority of patients presenting to the University Hospital of South Manchester with rectal carcinoma have not been diagnosed by the General Practitioner and occasionally have not been diagnosed by a consultant physician. Patients presenting with a right-sided colonic carcinoma often have rather non-specific symptoms of weight loss and anaemia and it is important that physicians recognise that these symptoms may be due to a colonic lesion and carry out the necessary investigation.

Treatment

Surgery is still the basis for treatment in most patients with colorectal carcinoma. In a select group of small tumours local excision may be justified, but usually a radical excision of the tumour with its lymphatic drainage area is undertaken (Fig. 7.2). In most cases the bowel continuity can be restored by anastomosis, but for very low rectal tumours a permanent end-colostomy is necessary after the radical excision (Fig. 7.3).

Although most large bowel carcinomas will show some regression with radiotherapy, this has little place as the primary treatment. It may be given as an adjuvant treatment either before or after operation for rectal tumour. The radiosensitivity of the tumour can be assessed by tissue culture of tumour cells with subsequent exposure to a standard dose of radiation (West *et al.*, 1989).

Chemotherapy is not of curative value in large bowel cancer. Unfortunately there is not, as yet, a satisfactory agent or combination. A meta-analysis of all published randomised trials of adjuvant chemotherapy shows no statistical difference between treated and control patients unless 5-fluorouracil (5-FU) was in the regime, when there was a minimal improvement in survival (Buyse *et al.*, 1988). This accords with the observation that 5-FU will reduce tumour bulk in 20 per cent of patients, but this is rarely of clinical usefulness (Moertel, 1978). Immunotherapy

Fig. 7.2. Operations for colon carcinoma. The broken outline indicates the area removed. (*a*) Right hemicolectomy. The small bowel at A is joined to the large bowel at B after the right half of the colon containing the tumour and a margin of normal bowel is removed together with its mesocolon and lymph nodes. (*b*) Left hemicolectomy. The large bowel at A is joined to the large bowel at B after the left half of the colon containing the tumour and a margin of normal tissue is removed with its associated lymph nodes and mesocolon. (*c*) Sigmoid colectomy. The large bowel at A is joined to the rectum at B after the sigmoid colon containing the tumour and a margin of normal tissue is removed with its associated lymph nodes and mesocolon.

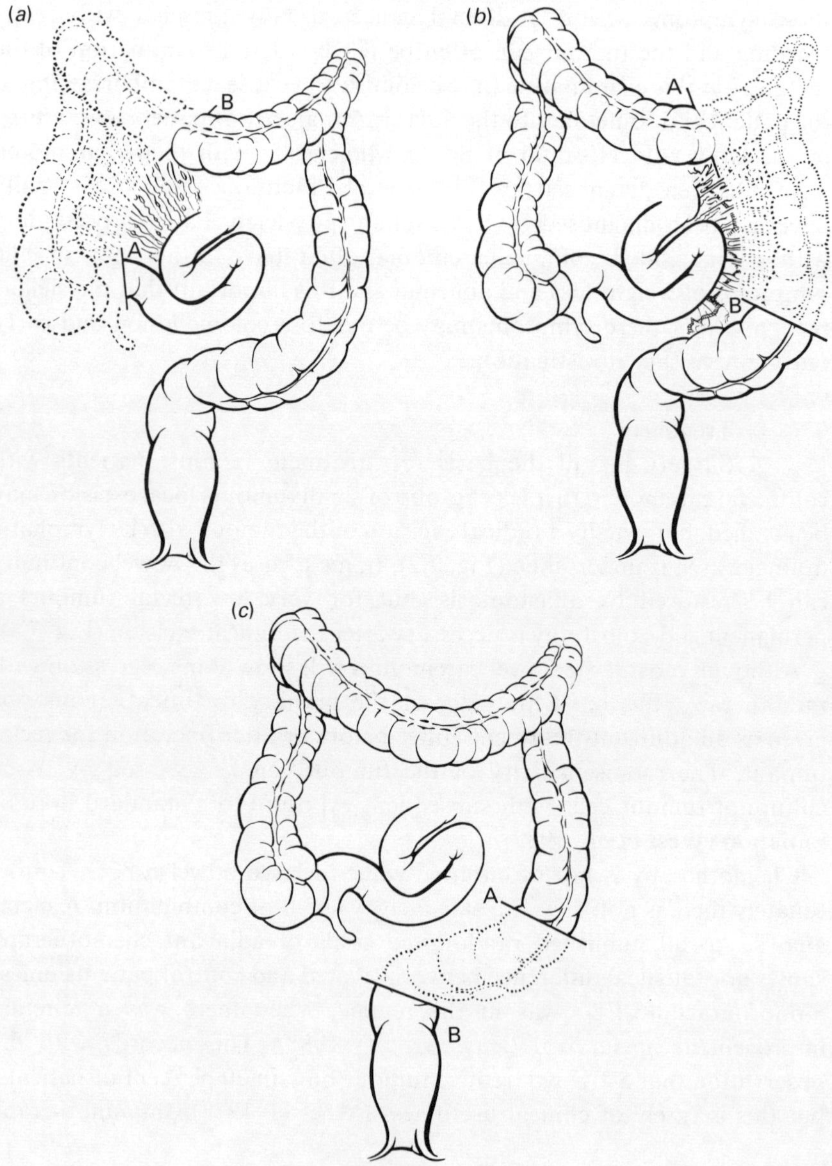

has not produced effective results either for advanced disease or in the adjuvant setting (Arnaud *et al.*, 1989). A recent study from the Mayo Clinic has shown some improvement in survival in Dukes' C colonic carcinoma patients by giving a combination of levamisole and 5-FU intermittently for 1 year after surgery (Laurie *et al.*, 1989). Immediate post-operative portal vein infusion of 5-FU may reduce the incidence of liver secondaries (Taylor *et al.*, 1985; Metzger, 1988). There have been suggestions that tagging a chemotherapeutic agent onto a monoclonal antibody will allow targeting of the chemotherapy; whilst this is attractive, it needs the discovery of a better agent before it can be exploited.

Post-operative screening

After the resection of a colorectal cancer it is usual to carry out regular post-operative surveillance. Several factors are germane: (1) colonic carcinomas may be multiple, (2) local recurrence may occur,

Fig. 7.3. Operations for rectal carcinoma. The broken outline indicates the area removed. (*a*) Anterior resection. The rectum is removed in part, including the tumour with a margin of normal tissue and the mesorectum and its associated lymph nodes, and the sigmoid colon at A joined to the lower rectum at B. (*b*) Abdomino-perineal resection. The whole of the rectum and anal canal containing the tumour is removed together with the mesorectum and associated lymph nodes. The cut end of the sigmoid colon at A is then brought through the abdominal wall as an end-colostomy.

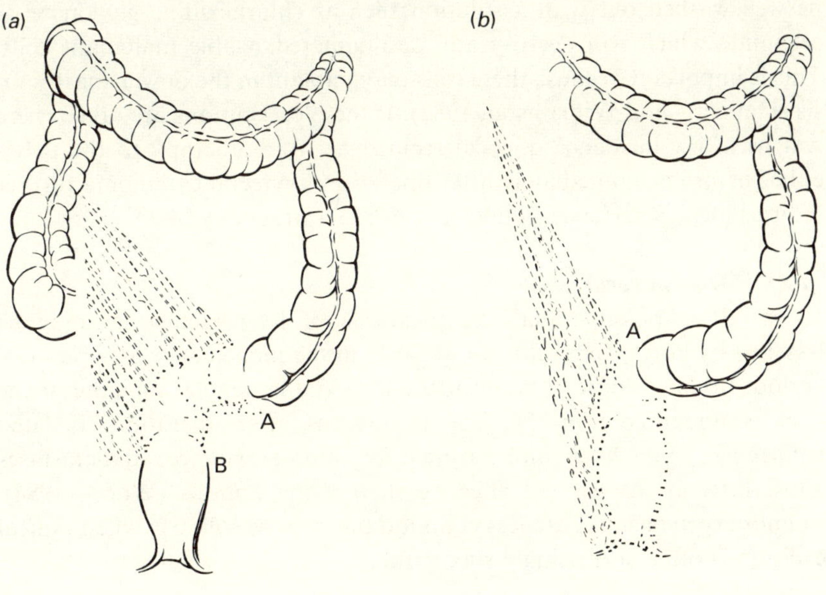

and (3) blood-borne metastases may occur, usually in the liver, occasionally in the lung and less frequently at other sites.

Multiple tumours

Ideally, the patient should have a total colonoscopy to assess the whole of the large bowel before operation because colorectal carcinoma may be multiple. A rate of synchronous colorectal carcinoma a little over 10 per cent has been reported from South Manchester (Cunliffe *et al.*, 1984). A tumour may make total preoperative colonoscopy impossible because it narrows the bowel to such an extent that the instrument cannot pass the narrowed area. Under these circumstances the colonoscopy should be done either at the time of the operation or a few weeks after the operation (Tate *et al.*, 1988). If the tumour is apparently curable and there is a second malignancy or multiple large adenomas, total colectomy and ileo-rectal anastomosis is probably the initial operation of choice (Fig. 7.1).

Local recurrence

Most local recurrence is due to inadequate excision of the primary tumour. This may be because of wide local spread at the time of operation making complete excision impossible but it may be due to inadequate surgery. This is particularly seen in the rectum, where it is important in order to prevent local recurrence to remove the mesorectum and wide lateral area (Heald *et al.*, 1982). In addition, the rectum should be well washed out with a solution such as chlorhexidine gluconate or cetrimide which will destroy any desquamated, viable malignant cells. This is important because these cells may implant in the bowel anastomosis (Umpleby and Williamson, 1987). If these precautions are taken there will be a low incidence of local recurrence. Radiotherapy to the pelvis either before or immediately after operation for rectal carcinoma further reduces local recurrence (Duncan, 1987; Gerard *et al.*, 1988).

Distant recurrence

It is possible that the incidence of liver metastases may be lessened by portal vein infusion of 5-FU in the immediate post-operative period. In an attempt to monitor the liver status, regular imaging of the liver is undertaken in the first 18 months after operation. Isolated recurrences in the liver can be excised for cure but widespread metastases allow little in the way of effective therapeutic options (Wood, 1984). Pulmonary metastases are less common but may be solitary, when radical excision is often surprisingly successful.

Second-look surgery

The surveillance of the post-operative patient is by the clinical and imaging modalities mentioned. In addition, CEA is measured regularly because if the disease recurs, CEA often becomes elevated before there is clinical evidence of recurrence. Unfortunately, it tends only to be elevated when there is a significant bulk of disease. It has been suggested that an elevation in the CEA level is an indication for a second-look laparotomy. This has been strongly advocated from the USA but it is rarely a useful stratagem because the recurrent tumour is usually irremovable. There is, at present, a national trial in progress in the UK which may resolve the usefulness of reoperation based on a raised CEA level (Northover, 1986).

Conclusions

The treatment of pre-malignant disease and its elimination is valuable in the prevention of colorectal cancer. Family histories may give a clue to high-risk groups which can be screened by colonoscopy. In the general population colonoscopy would not be indicated until the age of 50 years, but to perform colonoscopy on the whole of the relevant population is not feasible. For this reason a screening test is needed to reduce the number of colonoscopies required. The best available at the moment is the Hemoccult test for occult blood in the faeces, but this is imperfect. Population screening programmes on this basis do appear to have revealed cancer at an earlier stage but have not as yet shown any improvement in survival as a result of the earlier detection. Whether population screening is a cost-effective measure is open to argument. Education of both the population and medical practitioners about the early signs and symptoms of colonic disease is important because there is some evidence suggesting both patient and doctor delay in referring symptomatic patients for surgery.

The best treatment for colorectal cancer is surgery. In order that the surgery is appropriate it is important that the possibility of multiple colonic tumours is considered. In the light of this and the known areas of spread, the primary surgery should be radical in most cases. Adjuvant treatment by radiotherapy or portal vein chemotherapy may marginally improve survival. Surveillance of the patient post-operatively can occasionally find a curable recurrence but usually disease is incurable.

Better markers for colonic tumours are needed. Ideally these would be markers for adenoma which would allow the appropriate group to have colonoscopy and colonoscopic removal of adenoma in order to prevent the development of carcinoma.

References

Ahlquist, D. A. (1990) Colonic neoplasia: diagnosis and screening. *Curr. Opinion Gastroenterol.*, **6**, 33–7.

Arnaud, J. P., Buyse, M., Nordlinger, B., *et al.* (1989) Adjuvant therapy of poor prognosis colon cancer with levamisole: results of an EORTC double-blind randomised clinical trial. *Br. J. Surg.*, **76**, 284–9.

Bertario, L., Spindell, P., Gernari, L., *et al.* (1988) Sensitivity of Hemoccult test for large bowel cancer in high-risk subjects. *Dig. Dis. Sci.*, **33**, 609–13.

Blair, N. P. and Trempe, C. L. (1980) Hypertrophy of the retinal pigment epithelium associated with Gardner's syndrome. *Am. J. Ophthalmol.*, **90**, 661–7.

Buyse, M., Zeleniuch-Jacquotte, A. and Chalmers, T. C. (1988) Adjuvant therapy of colorectal cancer. *JAMA*, **259**, 3571–8.

Cunliffe, W. J., Hasleton, P. S., Tweedle, D. E. F. and Schofield P. F. (1984) Incidence of synchronous and metachronous colorectal carcinoma. *Br. J. Surg.*, **71**, 941–3.

Duncan, W. (1987) Preoperative radiotherapy in rectal cancer. *World J. Surg.*, **12**, 439–45.

Fujita, M., Sugiyama, R., Kumanishi, Y., *et al.* (1990) Evaluation of effectiveness of mass screening for colorectal cancer. *World J. Surg.*, **14**, 648–53.

Gerard, A., Buyse, M., Nordlinger, B., *et al.* (1988) Preoperative radiotherapy as adjuvant treatment of rectal cancer: final results of a randomised study of the European Organisation for Research and Treatment of Cancer (EORTC). *Ann. Surg.*, **208**, 606–14.

Gold, P. and Freedman, S. O. (1965) Demonstration of tumour specific antigens in human colonic carcinoma by immunological tolerance and absorption techniques. *J. Exp. Med.*, **121**, 439–62.

Grossman, S. and Milos, M. L. (1988) Colonoscopic screening of persons with suspected risk factors for colon cancer: family history. *Gastroenterology*, **94**, 395–400.

Hardcastle, J. D. and Pye, G. (1989) Screening for colorectal cancer: a critical view. *World J. Surg.*, **13**, 38–44.

Hardcastle, J. D., Chamberlain, J., Sheffield, J., *et al.* (1989) Randomised controlled trial of faecal occult blood screening for colorectal cancer: results for first 107,349 subjects. *Lancet*, **1**, 1160–4.

Heald, R. J., Husband, E. M., and Ryall, R. D. H. (1982) The mesorectum in rectal cancer surgery: the clue to pelvic recurrence? *Br. J. Surg.*, **69**, 613–16.

Hunter, R. D. (1989) Radiotherapy techniques. In: *The Causation and Clinical Management of Pelvic Radiation Disease*, ed. P. F. Schofield and E. W. Lupton, pp. 3–16. Springer, Berlin.

Itoh, H., Houlston, R. S., Haracopos, C. and Slack, J. (1990) Risk of cancer death in first-degree relatives of patients with hereditary non-polyposis cancer syndrome (Lynch type II): a study of 130 kindreds in the United Kingdom. *Br. J. Surg.*, **77**, 1367–70.

Jass, J. R. (1989) Do all colorectal carcinomas arise in preexisting adenomas? *World J. Surg.*, **13**, 45–51.

Knoepp, L. F. and McCulloch, J. H. (1978) Colonoscopy in the diagnosis of unexplained rectal bleeding. *Dis Colon Rectum*, **21**, 590–3.

Kronborg, O., Fenger, C., Sonergaard, O., *et al.* (1987) Initial mass screening for colorectal cancer with fecal occult blood test: a prospective randomised study at Funen in Denmark. *Scand J. Gastroenterol.*, **22**, 677–86.

Laurie, J. A., Moertel, C. G., Fleming, T.R., *et al.* (1989) Surgical adjuvant therapy of large bowel carcinoma: an evaluation of levamisole and the combination of levamisole and fluorouracil. The North Central Cancer Treatment Group and the Mayo Clinic. *J. Clin. Oncol.*, **7**, 1447–56.

Mandel, J. S., Bond, J. H., Bradley, M., *et al.* (1989) Sensitivity, specificity and positive predictivity of the Hemoccult test in screening for colorectal cancer: the University of Minnesota's colon cancer control study. *Gastroenterology*, **97**, 597–600.

Metzger, U. (1988) Intraportal chemotherapy for colorectal hepatic metastases. *Antibiot. Chemother.*, **40**, 51–60.

Moertel, C. G. (1976) Fluorouracil as an adjuvant to colorectal cancer surgery: the breakthrough that never was. *JAMA*, **236**, 1935–6.

Moore, M., Jones, D. J., Schofield, P. F. and Harnden, D. G. (1989) Current status of tumour markers in large bowel cancer. *World J. Surg.*, **13**, 52–9.

Morson, B. C. (1974) The polyp–cancer sequence in the large bowel. *Proc. R. Soc. Med.*, **67**, 451–7.

Northover, J. M. A. (1986) Carcinoembryonic antigen and recurrent colorectal cancer. *Gut*, **27**, 117–22.

Pye, G., Christie, M., Chamberlain, J., *et al.* (1988) A comparison of methods for increasing compliance with a general practitioner based screening project for colorectal cancer and the effect on practitioners' work load. *J. Epidemiol. Community Health*, **42**, 66–71.

Schofield, P. F. (1990) Colon, rectum and anus. In: *Cancer in the Elderly*, ed. F. I. Caird and T. B. Brewin, pp. 124–35. Wright, London.

Tate, J. J. T., Rawlinson, J., Royle, G. T., *et al.* (1988) Pre-operative or post-operative colonic examination for synchronous lesions in colorectal cancer. *Br. J. Surg.*, **75**, 1016–18.

Thoeni, R. F. and Menuck, L. (1977) Comparison of barium enema and colonoscopy in the detection of small colonic polyps. *Radiology*, **124**, 631–5.

Taylor, I., Machin, D., Mulle, M., *et al.* (1985) A randomized controlled trial of adjuvant portal vein cytotoxic perfusion in colorectal cancer. *Br. J. Surg.*, **72**, 359–63.

Umpleby, H. C. and Williamson, R. C. N. (1987) Anastomotic recurrence in large bowel cancer. *Br. J. Surg.*, **74**, 873–8.

West, C. M. L., Hunter, R. D., James, R. D. and Schofield, P. F. (1989) Surviving fractions at 2 Gray for colony-forming cells in primary culture of human cervical and colorectal tumours. *Symp. Proc. Am. Assoc. Physicists Med*, **7**, 86–95.

Wood, C. B. (1984) In: *Liver Metastases*, ed. E. J. H. Van de Velde and P. H. Sugarbaker, p. 47. Martinus Nijhoff, Amsterdam.

8

Future perspectives: Can the molecular biologist help the patient?

The development of colorectal carcinoma usually involves a step-wise progression from normal mucosa, through a benign adenoma, to a localised malignant stage and eventually a metastatic stage. Colorectal carcinoma is curable at any stage prior to the metastatic stage. Unfortunately, 20 per cent of patients who present already have obvious metastatic disease and eventually 60 per cent of all patients will succumb to metastatic disease.

As long as doctors have to wait for patients to present symptomatically with the disease, colorectal carcinoma will remain a major cause of death in developed countries. Strategies for its prevention must aim to avert the serious consequences of the disease by interrupting its natural progression. The success of such strategies depends on identifying the individuals at risk at either an asymptomatic early stage or prior to the metastatic phase, whilst the disease is still curable. As discussed in the previous chapter, those with an inherited predisposition can be screened by colonoscopy. There is a need for a screening test to select patients from the general population for colonoscopy, but to date no screening test, except for the presence of faecal occult blood (see Chapter 7), is clinically applicable in standard-risk patients.

The molecular biologist's view of the disease

Recently, specific genetic events associated with the progression of colorectal neoplasia have received much attention (Bodmer *et al.*, 1987; Bos *et al.*, 1987; Fearon *et al.*, 1987; Forrester *et al.*, 1987; Solomon *et al.*, 1987; Vogelstein *et al.*, 1988; Baker *et al.*, 1989; Fearon and Vogelstein, 1990; Bourne, 1991; Kinzler *et al.*, 1991). Colorectal tumours appear to arise from the mutational activation of oncogenes coupled to the loss or mutational inactivation of tumour suppressor genes. *Ras* gene mutations, and deletions and mutations of chromosome regions 5q, 17p and 18q, have been identified with the progression to localised malignancy. The specificity of the chromosomal losses (allelic deletions) has been interpreted as evidence that the regions affected contain tumour suppressor genes. Tumour suppressor genes are normal cellular genes the products of which regulate cellular growth and differentiation and inhibit the uncontrolled cellular proliferation associated with malignancy.

It has been suggested that these genes are recessive in that both copies of the gene must be lost or inactivated for uncontrolled growth to occur (Knudson, 1985; Hansen and Cavenee, 1987). However, the data are not entirely consistent with this thesis. Chromosomal and genetic analysis of adenomas from patients with FPC (FAP) does not reveal allelic losses of the 5q chromosomal region (Solomon *et al.*, 1987; Vogelstein *et al.*, 1988; Sasaki *et al.*, 1989). A study in Japan suggests that 5q allele loss is the second event and determines adenoma–carcinoma progression. The mutation in the other FPC (FAP) allele (the first event) is only permissive for the development of the adenoma (Miyaki *et al.*, 1990). This was recently confirmed with the identification of the gene for FPC (FAP) on chromosome region 5q21 (Bourne, 1991). Similarly in patients with inherited multiple endocrine neoplasia the wild-type allele on chromosome 10 does not appear to be lost in the tumour (Landsvater *et al.*, 1989; Nelkin *et al.*, 1989).

Fearon and Vogelstein (1990) proposed that these observations could be explained if some suppressor gene mutations effected a phenotypic change even in the presence of the wild-type allele. They selected p53, the gene loss associated with the 17p chromosomal deletions in colorectal carcinoma, as an example and reviewed the evidence, based on transfection studies in rodent cells, that a single mutated p53 could act as a dominant negative rather than a recessive mutation. It seemed likely, therefore, that in colorectal carcinoma a mutated p53 gene could provide a selective growth advantage leading to tumour progression. Detailed analysis of tumour samples has revealed that the subsequent loss of the wild-type allele is often associated with the progression from adenoma to carcinoma and an amplification of the effect provided by the initial mutation. Colorectal carcinomas with 17p allelic losses have been reported to be more aggressive than those without them (Kern *et al.*, 1989). It seems probable that other tumour suppressor genes implicated in colorectal carcinoma, such as the FAP gene, may also not conform to the classical recessive model (Bourne, 1991). Mutation in one allele may be sufficient to produce an altered cellular phenotype and progression of the disease, even in the presence of a wild-type allele – as in the case of p53.

Alternatively the level of expression of the protein product of some tumour suppressor genes may be critical and reduced expression of the product may alter some aspect of growth regulation. For example, the DCC gene on chromosome 18q codes for a cell adhesion molecule. A reduction in its expression in colorectal epithelial cells might lead to altered adhesion and a concomitant diminution of the associated growth-restraining signals (Fearon and Vogelstein, 1990).

Although Vogelstein and co-workers have demonstrated a preferred order for the accumulation of the genetic changes associated with colorectal malignancy, ultimately it is the accumulation rather than the order that is important (Chapter 6). However many genetic events are involved in colorectal tumour development, those identified so far provide a framework for the development of prognostic indicators. Fortunately, all the available evidence suggests that the molecular mechanisms involved are common to all forms of the disease, hereditary and non-hereditary.

Implications for screening strategies:

Although the genetic data are important, no tests have yet been devised which take advantage of them. The principal reason has been that information could only be obtained from adenoma and carcinoma specimens using detailed molecular biology techniques which did not lend themselves to rapid screening. Moreover, the numerous early histopathological studies using antibodies to identify *myc* and *ras* oncogene products were less than informative because the antibodies failed to distinguish between the mutant and wild-type gene products.

Nevertheless, increased knowledge of the specific genetic events associated with the progression to malignancy should present the possibility of early detection either by the identification of mutant gene products in the blood or faeces or through the detection of autoantibodies raised in the patient against the mutant gene products (Fearon and Vogelstein, 1990). These are not novel ideas, because in the case of colorectal tumours expression of the serum oncofetal protein carcinoembryonic antigen (CEA) has already been investigated as a tumour marker (Gold and Freedman, 1965; Colomer *et al.*, 1989; Imamura *et al.*, 1990) and antibodies directed against p53 in sera from breast cancer patients were described by Crawford *et al.* as long ago as 1982.

Anti-*ras* antibodies, however, fail to distinguish between the mutated and non-mutated protein products. Similarly mutations in p53 result in a protein with a prolonged half-life and in elevated levels of the protein product (easily detected by antibody staining and considered to be evidence of mutation), but until recently no distinction could be made between the mutated and non-mutated forms at the level of antibody detection. Patients are currently being screened for the production of mutant p53 antibodies (Vogelstein, American Association for the Advancement of Science, 1991).

Blood from patients with an inherited predisposition to FPC (FAP) could be screened at the DNA level for germ-line mutations and allelic loss on the long arm of chromosome 5 (5q21). Allelic loss of the p53 gene on chromosome region 17p (Baker *et al.*, 1989) is not unique to colorectal carcinoma, but is seen in more than 75 per cent of colorectal carcinomas (Vogelstein *et al.*, 1988; Delattre *et al.*, 1989) and has been associated with the progression of individual adenomas to carcinomas (Fearon *et al.*, 1987). Moreover, mutation in the other p53 allele has been shown to occur frequently in colorectal tumours (Baker *et al.*, 1989). These data were all obtained at the level of tumour cell DNA. Recently, however, germ-line transmission of a mutated p53 gene has been reported in cancer-prone families with Li-Fraumeni syndrome (Malkin *et al.*, 1990; Srivastava *et al.*, 1990), which means that only a blood sample is required from the patient. However, the usefulness of this observation remains in doubt as there are no real data on the frequency with which such an observation occurs and there are Li-Fraumeni patients with no evidence of a p53 mutation (Santibanez-Koref, Paterson Institute for Cancer Research, personal communication).

Screening for colorectal carcinoma in this country and worldwide is available to a very few due to external factors associated with patient management (availability of manpower and financial resources) and normally patients present symptomatically. For the most part, once the disease is established, i.e. recognisable as an adenoma or a carcinoma, the existing procedures for assessment are adequate. However, if we review the data presented above, there seem to be clear areas for the application of the genetic knowledge to the improved management of the disease. Individuals from families with FPC (FAP), Lynch's syndrome or simply a high incidence of colorectal carcinoma, can be screened early in life for FAP allele loss (and presumably mutation) and for p53 allele loss and mutation simply by taking a blood sample. Early detection of such changes could assist in the management and prevention of the disease on an individual basis. Similarly mutant gene products or antibodies to mutant gene products could be identified in blood serum as part of a general health screen.

Regarding the prognosis of established tumours, Birchmeier and co-workers have proposed that the expression of a 120 kDa cell-surface glycoprotein, E-cadherin (also known as Arc-1, uvomorulin, and cell-CAM 120/80), might act as a marker of invasive potential and metastasis (Frixen *et al.*, 1991). Examination of human bladder, breast and lung carcinoma cell lines exhibiting various degrees of differentiation and invasion as assessed by *in vitro* assays, showed reduced E-cadherin expression as assessed by fluorescent staining and western and northern blot analysis to correlate with increased invasiveness and poor differentiation. The human E-cadherin gene is located on chromsome 16q22.1 (Natt *et al.*, 1989), which is exactly the location of a putative suppressor gene for human hepatocellular carcinoma (Tsuda *et al.*, 1990) and possibly prostate cancer (Carter *et al.*, 1990). It may be, therefore, that E-cadherin is another candidate for a tumour suppressor gene, although allelic losses on the long arm of chromosome 16 are rare in colorectal carcinomas (Fearon and Vogelstein, 1990). The gene has been cloned and monoclonal antibodies raised to the human E-cadherin gene product (Frixen *et al.*, 1991) which are currently being used in the author's laboratory to screen clinical samples of colonic tissue in frozen section (Kinsella *et al.*, unpublished observations). E-cadherin expression is also being studied in established colorectal carcinoma cell lines with a view to correlating its expression with the behaviour of the cell lines in *in vitro* and *in vivo* experimental models of metastasis. If a reduction in or absence of E-cadherin expression can be correlated with the metastatic phenotype it becomes a very important prognostic indicator, not only because fluorescein-tagged antibody staining should be easy to execute at the time of routine pathology but also because a significant number of colorectal carcinomas that appear to only be locally invasive at the time of resection go on to metastasise. If this subgroup could be identified at the time of surgery the subsequent patient management could be different.

The DCC gene product, a cell adhesion molecule, might be a useful marker of tumour progression. It is certain that in tumours where *ras*, p53 and DCC gene mutations are not identified, other as yet unknown genes must be effecting equivalent changes in phenotype. Identification of the missing molecular steps by the scientist can only help to facilitate better patient management and a better clinical outcome for the disease. Thus, carcinoma of the colon, singled out by research scientists for special attention because of its clear step-wise progression, looks like providing the key to our understanding of the development of several common solid tumours. This should lead to a concomitant improvement in screening and treatment strategies for malignancy in general.

References

Baker, S. J., Fearon, E. R., Nigro, J. M., *et al.* (1989) Chromosome 17 deletions and p53 gene mutations in colorectal carcinomas. *Science*, **244**, 217–21.

Bodmer, W. F., Bailey, C. J., Bodmer, J., *et al.* (1987) Localisation of the gene for familial adenomatous polyposis on chromsome 5. *Nature*, **328**, 614–16.

Bos, J. L., Fearon, E. R., Hamilton, S. R., *et al.* (1987) Prevalence of *ras* gene mutations in colorectal cancers. *Nature*, **327**, 293–7.

Bourne, H. R. (1991) Suppression with a difference. *Nature*, **353**, 696–8.

Carter, B. S., Ewing, C. M., Ward, W. S., *et al.* (1990) Allelic losses of chromosomes 16q and 10q in human prostate cancer. *Proc. Natl. Acad. Sci. USA*, **87**, 8751–5.

Colomer, R., Ruibal, A. and Salvador, L. (1989) Circulating tumour marker levels in advanced carcinoma correlate with the extent of metastatic disease. *Cancer*, **64**, 1674–81.

Crawford, L. V., Pim, D. C. and Bulbrook, R. D. (1982) Detection of antibodies against the cellular protein p53 in sera from patients with breast cancer. *Int. J. Cancer*, **30**, 403–8.

Delattre, P., Olschwang, S., Law, D., *et al.* (1989) Multiple genetic alterations distinguish distal from proximal colorectal cancer. *Lancet*, **2**, 353–6.

Fearon, E. R. and Vogelstein, B. (1990) A genetic model for colorectal tumourigenesis. *Cell*, **61**, 759–67.

Fearon, E. R., Hamilton, S. R. and Vogelstein, B. (1987) Clonal analysis of human colorectal tumours. *Science*, **238**, 193–7.

Forrester, K., Almoguera, C., Han, K., *et al.* (1987) Detection of high incidence of K-*ras* oncogenes during human colon tumourigenesis. *Nature*, **327**, 298–303.

Frixen, U. H., Behrens, J., Sachs, M., *et al.* (1991) E-cadherin-mediated cell–cell adhesion prevents invasiveness of human carcinoma cells. *J. Cell Biol.*, **113**, 173–85.

Gold, P. and Freedman, S. O. (1965) Demonstration of tumour-specific antigens in human colon carcinomata by immunological tolerance and absorption techniques. *J. Exp. Med.*, **121**, 439–62.

Hansen, M. F. and Cavenee, W. K. (1987) Genetics of cancer predisposition. *Cancer Res.*, **47**, 5518–27.

Imamura, Y., Yasutake, K., Yoshimura, Y., *et al.*, (1990) Contents of tissue CEA and CA19-9 in colonic polyp and colorectal cancer and their clinical significance. *Gastroenterol. Jpn.*, **25**, 186–92.

Kern, S. E., Fearon, E. R., Tersmette, K. W. F., *et al.* (1989) Clinical and pathologic associations with allelic loss in colorectal carcinoma. *JAMA*, **261**, 3099–103.

Kinzler, K. W., Nilbert, M., Vogelstein, B., *et al.* (1991) Identification of a gene located at chromosome 5q21 that is mutated in colorectal cancers. *Science*, **251**, 1366–70.

Knudson, A. G. (1985) Hereditary cancer, oncogenes and anti-oncogenes. *Cancer Res.*, **45**, 1437–43.

Landsvater, R. M., Mathew, C. G. P., Smith, B. A., *et al.* (1989) Development of multiple endocrine neoplasia type 2A does not involve substantial deletions of chromsome 10. *Genomics*, **4**, 246–50.

Malkin, D., Li, F. P., Strong, L. C., *et al.* (1990) Germ line p53 mutations in a familial syndrome of breast cancer, sarcomas and other neoplasms. *Science*, **250**, 1233–8.

Miyaki, M., Seki, M., Okamoto, M., *et al.* (1990) Genetic changes and histopathological types in colorectal tumours from patients with Familial Adenomatous Polyposis. *Cancer Res.*, **50**, 7166–73.

Natt, E., Magenis, R. E., Zimmer, J., *et al.* (1989) Regional assignment of the human loci for uvomorulin (UVO) and chymotrypsinogen B (CTRB) with the help of two overlapping deletions on the long-arm of chromsome 16. *Cytogenet. Cell Genet.*, **50**, 145–8.

Nelkin, B. D., Nakamura, Y., White, R. W., *et al.* (1989) Low incidence of loss of chromosome 10 in sporadic and hereditary human medullary thyroid carcinoma. *Cancer Res.*, **49**, 4114–19.

Sasaki, M., Okamoto, M., Sato, C., *et al.* (1989) Loss of constitutional heterozygosity in colorectal tumours from patients with familial polyposis coli and those with non-polyposis colorectal carcinoma. *Cancer Res.*, **49**, 4402–6.

Sherlock, P., Lipkin, M. and Winawer, S. J. (1980) The prevention of colon cancer: a combined clinic and basic science seminar. *Am. J. Med.*, **68**, 917–31.

Solomon, E., Voss, R., Hall, V., *et al.* (1987) Chromosome 5 allele loss in colorectal carcinomas. *Nature*, **328**, 616–19.

Srivastava, S., Zou, Z., Pirollo, K., *et al.* (1990) Germ-line transmission of a mutated p53 gene in a cancer-prone family with Li-Fraumeni syndrome. *Nature*, **348**, 747–9.

Tsuda, H., Zhang, W., Shimosato, Y., *et al.* (1990) Allele loss on chromosome 16 associated with progression of human hepatocellular carcinoma. *Proc. Natl. Acad. Sci. USA*, **87**, 6791–4.

Vogelstein, B., Fearon, E. R., Hamilton, S. R., *et al.* (1988) Genetic alterations during colorectal tumour development. *New Engl. J. Med.*, **319**, 525–32.

Vogelstein, B., Fearon, E. R., Kern, S. E., *et al.* (1989) Allelotype of colorectal carcinomas. *Science*, **244**, 207–11.

Index